Praise for *Ayurveda Cooking for Beginners*

"In *Ayurveda Cooking for Beginners*, Laura Plumb has made the profound knowledge of Ayurvedic nutrition accessible to everyone. As you enjoy her many creative recipes, you will also learn how food can balance your own individual mind-body constitution and support you in optimal wellness."

DR. DAVID FRAWLEY, Vedacharya and author of *Yoga & Ayurveda*

"Hippocrates said 'Let food be thy medicine, and medicine be thy food.' In *Ayurveda Cooking for Beginners*, Laura Plumb makes it such a joy to create delicious, healing meals that one's relationship with food is forever transformed."

MELANIE FIORELLA, MD, Associate Clinical Professor of Integrative Health at UC San Diego and visiting staff member of the Chopra Center's Mind-Body Medical Group

"As Director of the Kerala Ayurveda Academy, I have personally witnessed Laura's profound understanding of the deeper principles of Ayurvedic wellness. *Ayurveda Cooking for Beginners* should have a central place in the kitchens of everyone desiring a healthier, happier life."

DR. JAYRAJAN KODIKKANATH, Ayurvedic doctor and Director of Kerala Ayurveda Clinics and Academy

"Laura has made it easy and enjoyable to bring the healing science of Ayurveda into your kitchen and enjoy delicious nutrition. You will be healthier, your family will thrive, and my prediction is there will be fewer visits to the doctor!"

DR. RAMKUMAR KUTTY, founder and director of the Vaidyagrama Ayurveda Healing Community

"I'm in love with this book—and Laura Plumb! She is an example of the awakened Divine Feminine. *Ayurveda Cooking for Beginners* is a delightful guide to supporting and nourishing the health and well-being of powerful women. Laura has created a way for us to grow our 'balance-arsenal' of foods that bring rejuvenation, energy, and vibrancy. In this book, Laura shows what is possible in the realm of holistic wellness."

HEMALAYAA, Transformation Facilitator and Leadership Coach

"Laura Plumb inspires others to achieve vitality and radiant health. *Ayurveda Cooking for Beginners* should be on everyone's bookshelf because understanding the principals of Ayurveda is essential to health and wellness."

MELISSA AMBROSINI, bestselling author & speaker

"Absolutely delicious book! *Ayurveda Cooking for Beginners* is a beautiful guidebook that brings awareness of healthy foods and fosters a love for cooking."

DR. MANISHA KSHIRSAGAR, BAMS, co-founder and co-director of the Ayurvedic Healing Clinic in Santa Cruz, CA, and author of *Enchanting Beauty*

Ayurveda Cooking for Beginners

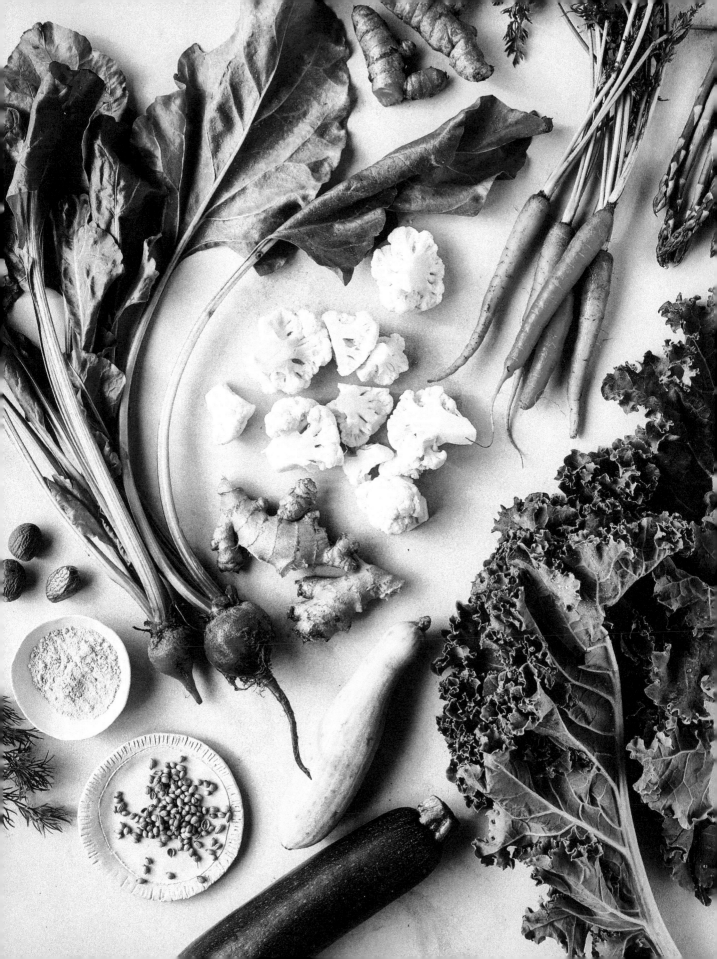

Ayurveda Cooking

for Beginners

An Ayurvedic Cookbook to Balance & Heal

Laura Plumb

Photography by Hélène Dujardin

R

ROCKRIDGE
PRESS

For general information on our other products and services or to obtain
technical support, please contact our Customer Care Department within
the United States at (866) 744-2665, or outside the United States
at (510) 253-0500.

Rockridge Press publishes its books in a variety of electronic and print
formats. Some content that appears in print may not be available in
electronic books, and vice versa.

TRADEMARKS: Rockridge Press and the Rockridge Press logo are trademarks or registered trademarks of Callisto Media Inc. and/or its affiliates,
in the United States and other countries, and may not be used without
written permission. All other trademarks are the property of their respec-
tive owners. Rockridge Press is not associated with any product or vendor
mentioned in this book.

Photography © Hélène Dujardin/Food styling by Lisa Rovick

ISBN: Print 978-1-62315-963-4 | eBook 978-1-62315-964-1

For Morgan,
my first student
of Ayurveda and
an always-willing
recipe taster.

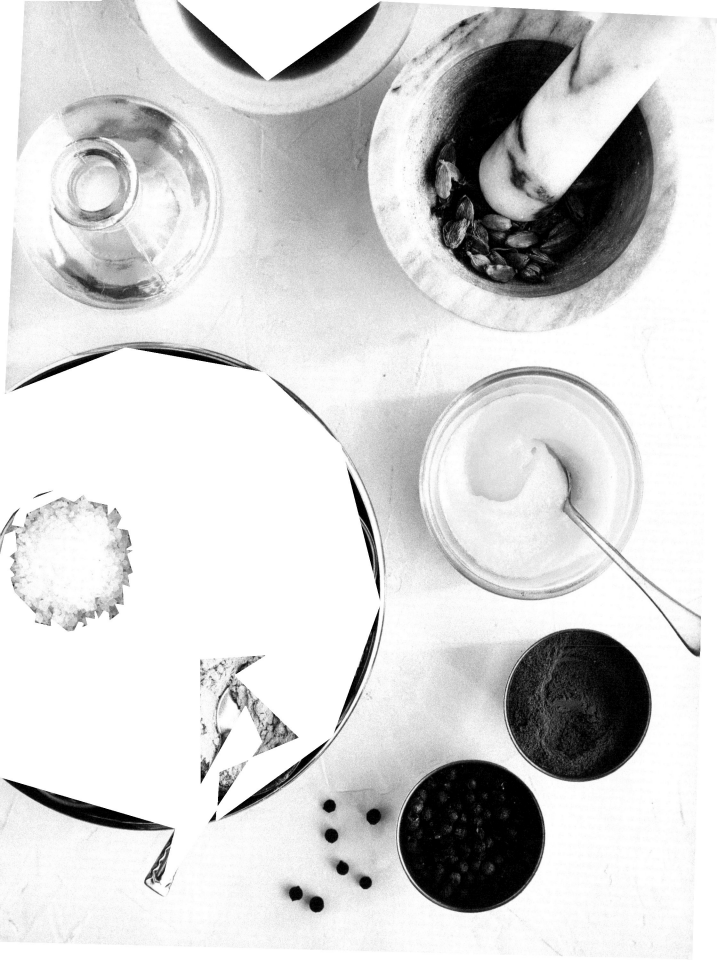

Contents

Introduction **x**

part one Your Ayurvedic Primer 1

one Core Concepts in Ayurveda 3

two Ayurveda & Food 25

three Five Steps to Ayurvedic Eating 41

part two Recipes to Balance & Heal 53

four Staples & Spices 57

five Teas & Tonics 71

six Breakfasts 83

seven Hearty & Satisfying Lunches 97

eight Light & Simple Dinners 119

nine Ayurvedic Spins on Favorites 143

ten Soothing Savories & Sweets 159

eleven Condiments, Spreads & Sauces 173

Appendix A: An In-Depth Look at Doshic States 189

Appendix B: Seasonal & Dosha-Balancing Food Lists 197

Appendix C: The Substances of Our Universe 202

The Dirty Dozen & the Clean Fifteen 203

Resources 204

Season & Dosha Recipe Index 207

Recipe Index 212

Index 214

Introduction

I REMEMBER LONG SUMMER NIGHTS when as children we would lay ourselves out on the grass and gaze up into the vast night sky. Do you remember that excitement and wonder? It was as if your whole body was listening while you felt the whole world glistening.

Subsequently in my life I found a science that articulates this experience. It's called Ayurveda, and it's a comprehensive system of healing and wellness that arises from the universal wisdom embodied in this quote from its ancient Sanskrit roots, *Yatha pinde tatha brahmande*:

In the microcosm is the macrocosm. In the atom is the cosmos.
In the personal is the universal. In the one is the all.

Ayurveda is a tangible reminder that you are an integral part of this natural world, alive with radiance and grace. In fact, you are a mirror of all that is mighty and majestic, and you are made of the very same power that ignites and sustains all existence.

From the root words *Ayur* meaning "life," and *Veda* meaning "science," Ayurveda does not define a person by their illness. Instead it views each individual as a vital expression of life, with intelligence and regenerative powers that sometimes need support and nurturing. In this way, Ayurveda restores dignity to patients and humanity to medicine.

Its service to the wider world is in its simple, easy-to-adopt, and intuitive systems for better living—and those joys start in the kitchen. According to the *Charak Samhita*, an ancient Ayurvedic text:

The distinction between health and disease arises as the result of the difference between wholesome and unwholesome diet.

To me, cooking is where Ayurvedic wisdom comes home, where nature, in her great generosity, offers herself most fully to us—letting us touch, taste, smell, and behold her bounty while turning everyday meals into delights of nourishing balance and healing.

I began writing about Ayurvedic cooking to support the health of family, friends, and clients: to nourish a teenager, rejuvenate a grandmother, soothe the digestive issues of a brother, calm the anxiety of a bereaved mother, and strengthen the bones and organs of a husband whose journalistic career left his body ravaged from covering wars.

As a practitioner of Ayurvedic medicine, I have witnessed people over the years transform their lives by changing their relationship with food. I have seen the power of pure grains, organic vegetables, juicy fruits, and natural spices to ignite recovery, renew passion, foster hope, and exalt purpose.

Over the years, the question I hear most often is how to simplify Ayurveda and interpret it for busy modern lives and families. This book is an answer to that question. It offers:

- An overview of Ayurvedic concepts simple enough to apply right away.
- Handy tables and lists to make shopping, cooking, and eating according to the principles of Ayurveda convenient, affordable, and delicious.
- Delicious, easy recipes, usually using no more than five primary ingredients and some seasoning or spices.
- Suggestions and tips for every recipe to suit all dosha types, budgets, and lifestyles.

Ayurvedic cooking is a sumptuous blend of science, art, love, and nourishment. It unlocks nature's healing power and connects you to the inherent wisdom already within you. As you read this book, learn these concepts, and begin to cook Ayurvedically, it's likely you will experience what I call the *full body nod*–that gentle rocking sway that comes when every part of you sings "Yay!"

In reality, this book is just a reminder of what you already know somewhere deep within. It is a wisdom that has been transmitted through families for generations, and it is a wisdom that we cannot afford to lose. Our world, and all of us in it, needs Ayurveda now more than ever.

In this era of devastating diet-related illnesses, I passionately feel that we must remind people that eating for health can be a simple, sacred, and sumptuous delight. While this book is but a taste of Ayurveda's fullest reach, I hope it is a taste that satisfies, nourishes, and inspires you to learn more.

part one | Your Ayurvedic Primer

The ancient science of Ayurveda is really *the art of living wisely,* as it empowers people to make choices that nurture and sustain the body and the mind for optimal wellness. As a science that harnesses the healing intelligence within nature, Ayurveda bases its wisdom on the five elements present everywhere in existence: space, air, fire, water, and earth.

Understanding the five elements and their properties gives you access to one of the world's most elegant and integrated methods of healing and peak living. Empowering you with simple, easy-to-understand tools, Ayurveda cultivates your inner intelligence to support the best of you, the blossoming of health, radiance, beauty, and heart, while empowering greater fulfillment in all areas of life.

Through Ayurveda, we become the masters of our own lives, living its wisdom artfully.

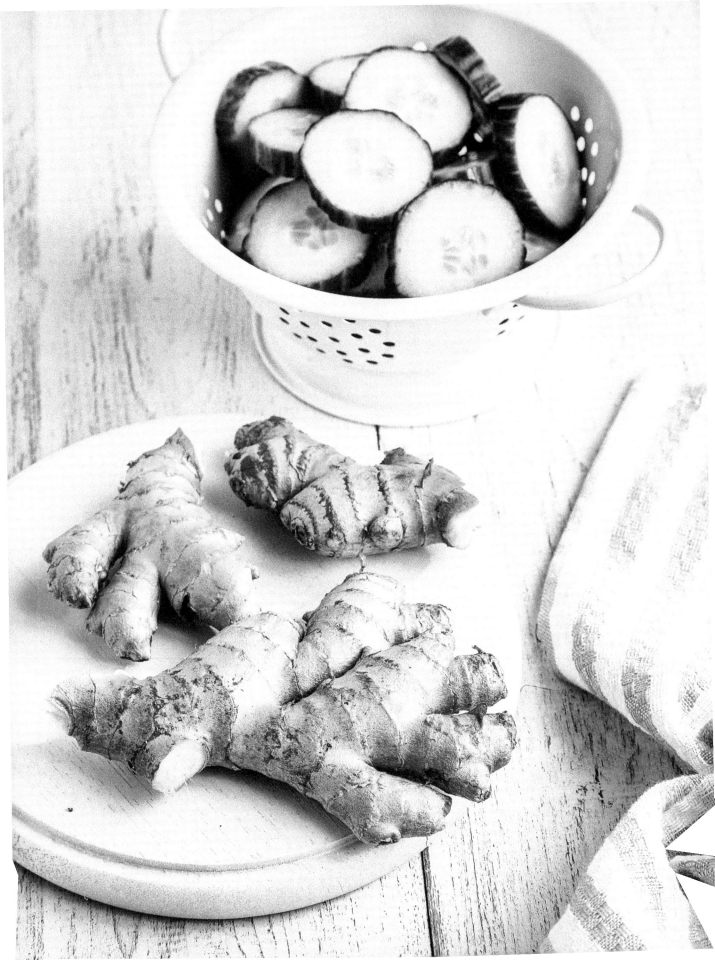

one
Core Concepts in Ayurveda

Some of you have watched a flower winding up a string, a morning glory winding around a string. Perhaps you have seen a vine climbing up a lattice, and you have watched the end coming out, and turning in, back and forth, between the interstices of the lattice. How does the vine know what to do? There is an intelligence that is present in the plant, in all vegetation.

—JOHN HARVEY KELLOGG

An Ancient Science

Ayurveda is considered the oldest comprehensive system of medicine in the world, with roots possibly going all the way back to the 50,000-year-old spiritual healing technology of shamanism. As a systematic body of healing knowledge, Ayurveda arose during the Vedic Sarasvati culture that flourished in the western Himalayan plains from around 7000 BCE to about 1900 BCE.

Often referred to as the "mother of all healing," Ayurveda is believed to have spread with Buddhism through most of Asia, where it intermixed with traditional Chinese medicine, and then headed westward with trade, influencing the Hippocratic medicine of Greece.

Ayurveda inherits the fundamental principle that there is a subjective, knowable reality, an awareness or pure consciousness, underlying all existence.

This underlying consciousness is an intelligence that animates all life. We are aware of this in our own human existence through our perception, our capacity to see, feel, hear, smell, taste, and experience the world.

From Ayurveda's origins comes the concept that consciousness gives rise to existence and embeds itself within life, with the power to generate and regenerate life. This tremendous insight, that consciousness is the healer, means that any living organism in a state of equilibrium has the capacity to naturally and spontaneously heal itself.

For this reason, equilibrium or homeostasis, what we usually refer to as *balance*, is key to Ayurvedic healing. This is not the same as the restrictive notion of "moderation in all things." Instead, Ayurveda helps us conduct the symphonic interplay of the dynamic forces of nature, tuning ourselves as instruments, exalting in the song of life.

Ayurveda for Modern Life

In a world where stress is the primary cause of disease, Ayurveda reminds us of our aliveness, humanity, inner power, intelligence, and inherent peace. It reconnects us to a world that pulses with light, sings with sumptuous beauty, and nourishes with delight. Its time-tested wisdom has never been more important and valuable than in our modern times.

Ayurveda Is a Root Medicine

Ayurveda is at the historic root of medical systems, and it fundamentally seeks to dissolve the root cause of disease to reestablish the natural state of well-being.

In our modern world, medical treatment tends to focus on medications to relieve our symptoms rather than to address the underlying conditions. Ayurveda liberates us from the dangers of a multitude of pharmaceutical side effects, instead cultivating optimal health and wellness through positive lifestyle changes that include diet, exercise, and emotional well-being—whether one is recovering from a grave illness or simply seeking greater clarity and vitality.

Ayurveda Restores Humanity to Medicine

Ayurveda is a nature-based approach to healing that recognizes the unique difference of every individual and that, because every one of us is unique, *every illness or imbalance is unique*. In Ayurveda, we seek to treat *the whole person*, by attempting to understand each individual's constitution, circumstances, lifestyle, tastes, habits, thoughts, attitude, and relationships.

Ayurveda Is Accessible

Given that Ayurveda treats individuals differently, if 10 people have the same disease, there will be 10 different treatments. With more than 7 billion people alive now, this suggests that Ayurveda has 7 billion potential treatments.

In fact, Ayurveda is a complex system, with a great variety of tools for healing. But it is based on the simple principles of the five elements of nature, which are knowable and accessible to all. Its modalities involve lifestyle changes, dietary adaptations, and inexpensive herbs and herbal formulas, and often these modalities include no-cost interventions like meditation, prayer, exercise, and sleep enhancement.

Ayurveda Is Empowering

Through its many accessible tools, Ayurveda supports your own healing power. Whether it is by learning about your dosha, how to prepare meals to achieve balance, or techniques to promote relaxation, self-esteem grows with every incremental accomplishment. As a result, your body's healing powers strengthen. It is uplifting to find this capacity within ourselves, and that empowers our resolve to continue.

Ayurveda Feels Good

Love makes you feel vibrant. Happiness puts a spring in your step. Peace of mind gives you comfort, confidence, and the clarity to make the right choices.

Ayurveda understands that how you feel emotionally affects how you feel physically, as well as the choices you make, so it has tools to address mental and emotional balance. Ultimately, Ayurveda is so much more than a science seeking the absence of disease: Ayurveda supports the best and fullest expression of your most radiant being.

The Importance of Paying Attention

Beyond promoting health, Ayurveda asks us to look at what we do with our health, energy, and longevity. This scrutiny requires attention and self-inquiry. With proper attention to our surroundings and their effect on us, we make better choices. Through self-inquiry, we understand, nourish, and express ourselves with greater authenticity, compassion, and creativity.

Here are five practical ways to cultivate a refined awareness that makes Ayurvedic living intuitive and simple:

1. **Observe your breath.** As you take a deep breath, notice how it feels. Notice as you pause and hold that breath. As you exhale, where do you feel your breath releasing?

2. **Notice sensations.** Bring all your attention to the top of your head, and notice any sensations as you slowly scan your entire body. Scan the right side, the left side, your front and back, all the way down to your feet, and then back up to the top of your head.

3. **Focus your five senses.** Take a soft gaze and gently observe the light, shadows, colors, and shapes in your environment. Listen to the sounds around you—outer/inner, loud/soft, gentle/grating. Shift your attention to the aromas floating by. Close your eyes and see if that makes the aromas stronger, more distinct. Continue this with the sense of touch, and then taste. Practice bringing your fullest attention to your senses through-out the day.

4. **Be curious about the qualities within and around you.** Observe the way you feel right now. Do you feel hot or cold? Heavy or light? Can you imagine feeling the opposite? Does that bring balance? What are the qualities in your environment right now? Clear or foggy? Wet? Dry? See page 202 for more on the qualities of nature.

5. **Pause and listen.** Ask yourself, *What am I sensing right now?* Listen to the answer. Pause long enough for the quieter aspects within you to rise up in response. Sometimes it helps to ask a few times. *What am I feeling right now?* There are no right or wrong answers. There is only information, hopefully wisdom, and ultimately greater self-care.

As you play with these practices, simply witness, releasing any tendency to look for an answer or to achieve a "correct" way of doing it. Observe in the same way you might watch a baby giggle, sleep, or take her first steps. Allow yourself to be curious and fully embrace whatever is there to be perceived.

The Three Vital Essences of Ayurveda

Ayurveda is enlivening because it gives you permission to be wholly and uniquely you. It affirms what you intuitively know about yourself. It aligns you with the rhythms of nature in a way that feels mystical and magical, yet authentic and integrated.

Prana, Tejas, Ojas

You are a healing power, a regenerative genius, an intelligent being alive with unique talents, beauty, and gifts. There is no one like you, and there is no science as dedicated as Ayurveda to nurturing that uniqueness, to enhancing the power and the glory of you.

What makes you so individually unique, yet an integral part of the whole at the same time?

It's the same thing that makes the world go round—a power Ayurvedic sages called *prana*, *tejas*, and *ojas*. These Sanskrit words for dynamism, radiance, and cohesion, respectively, are the underlying forces of existence. In the cosmos, *prana* is electromagnetism, *tejas* is thermodynamics, and *ojas* is gravity. In nature, *prana* is aliveness, *tejas* is intelligence, and *ojas* is wholeness and integrity. In the individual, *prana* is life energy, *tejas* is digestion and metabolism, and *ojas* is lubrication and structure.

When *prana* is strong, you have creativity, curiosity, agility, quickness of mind and movement, lightness of heart, a healing touch, and the capacity to listen well. When *tejas* is strong, you have radiance, enthusiasm, clarity, courage, focus, discernment, determination, leadership, a good sense of humor, and positive passion. When *ojas* is strong, you have peace, patience, contentment, kindness, nurturance, connection, endurance, resilience, longevity, stamina, strength, and stability.

Prana, *tejas*, and *ojas* are the positive impulses of life, found everywhere in nature. When our *prana*, *tejas*, and *ojas* are strong, we have balance, energy, intelligence, and integrity. We feel grounded yet vibrantly alive. We feel stable yet active. We rest and digest well, and we respond powerfully, clearly, and spontaneously to the needs of each moment.

Prana is life's capacity to think, feel, move, create, generate, and regenerate. *Tejas* is light, heat, and fire. It helps us see what's real, discern truth, digest experience, and burn away all that is impure or illusory. *Ojas* is lubricating, grounding, protecting, and immune building. It is said to be the product of digestion and metabolism, stored as golden drops of nectar in the heart.

In the natural world, *prana* gives wind that propels weather and carries the seeds of life. *Tejas* is fire giving warmth that cleanses and transforms. *Ojas* is water, where molecules unite to give rise to new life and growth occurs.

In the broadest sense, *prana* is life, *tejas* is light, and *ojas* is love.

Balancing these forces gives radiant health. Increasing these forces gives presence, wisdom, and compassion. Ayurvedic cooking cultivates these powers through dynamically balanced meals that nourish your energy, intelligence, and strength to bring out the best in you.

The Five Elements of the Universe

In the beginning was the word … into a vast, dark space, vibration arises. From that first wave of sound comes movement. Movement causes friction. Friction creates heat and suddenly erupts into fire. A star is born. In that star, and all other stars, chemical reactions occur. Hydrogen, helium, oxygen, carbon, iron … the periodic table emerges. The fire burns bright. The heat becomes too great. The star explodes, scattering molecules of future life across the sky. Eventually these molecules are drawn together by a mystery referred to as gravity. Hydrogen and oxygen bind and become water. Water attracts and coheres. More molecules adhere. Multicelled life appears. Slowly our planet Earth grows trees, plants, flowers, fish, birds, animals, and humans.

Ayurveda explains that we are each microcosms of the macrocosm–the universe within each being–and that you are whole, the totality of all, a dynamic play of swirling energies, radiant light, and complex intelligence. The universe of which we are each an integral part is made up of five prime elements: space, air, fire, water, and earth. These elements, alone and in combination, are found everywhere in nature, including in you and in every human being.

The Three Doshas

What makes each of us unique is the individual combination of these elements. One person may have all five elements more or less evenly balanced. Another may have a high predominance of one element over the others. Someone else may have two elements predominant.

The tendency of an element to be dominant is called a dosha. *Dosha* is a Sanskrit word at the root of our English word *dysfunction*. It refers to the tendency of a living organism to become imbalanced due to the persistent dominance of elements.

In excess, the air or space elements create a Vata dosha. Pitta is excess of the fire element combined with water–much like acidic gastric juices. Excess water or earth turns the nectar of *ojas* into the imbalance of Kapha.

In Vedic philosophy, the five elements emerge from the three vital essences of *prana*, *tejas*, and *ojas*: You could say that the doshas are the imbalanced state of space, air, fire, water, and earth, while *prana*, *tejas*, and *ojas* are the correct functioning of those elements within: space and air from *prana*, fire from *tejas*, and water and earth from *ojas*.

Spend time in nature: The Ayurvedic sages spent their entire lives observing nature. Spending time outside helps you absorb nature's medicine and become attuned to the intelligence of the elements and the dynamics of the doshas.

In health, *prana* gives good circulation, energy, proper functioning of all physiological systems, and alert mental and cognitive functions. *Tejas* gives strong digestion and a capacity to convert food to energy, to burn off toxins, and to purify tissue. It also gives mental clarity, radiance, and courage. *Ojas* gives well-formed tissue, lubrication in the joints, comfort, strength, and good immune function.

What we seek to do through Ayurveda is to reduce, pacify, or balance our doshas. We never increase a dosha—that would increase a dysfunction or imbalance. Instead, through intelligent balance we restore the positive state of *prana*, *tejas*, and *ojas* to stimulate a natural surge of healing and regeneration.

VATA

Prana expresses in nature as air and space, which give Vata light, mobile, and dry qualities. Vata can make one feel spacey, scattered, or restless. There can be insomnia or anxiety, with physical conditions like joint pain, cold feet, constipation, tremors, arthritis, weakness, chronic fatigue, and degenerative bone and neurological disorders.

PITTA

Fire emerges from the subtle essence of *tejas*, which is light and dry, but Pitta dosha combines fire with some water, so its qualities are hot, sharp, light, and liquid or oily. Pitta can give rise to irritability, impatience, anger, indigestion, and liver disorders. There might be skin issues such as rashes, acne, boils, or, more seriously, chronic inflammation, hypertension, and heart disease.

KAPHA

Ojas gives structure and stability through the elements of earth and water, which give Kapha the qualities of wet, cool, and heavy. Kapha dosha can give sluggishness, sadness, a lack of motivation, depression, and even greed or too much attachment to people and things. Physically, Kapha may be prone to asthma, seasonal allergies, chronic congestion, obesity, diabetes, and cancer.

The Three Doshas

Throughout my years of working with students and clients, I've found that they enjoy learning about their dosha and through that come to a greater understanding of their particular strengths and energetic tendencies. This is a simplified quiz to help you determine your predominant dosha. If two answers apply, either choose the one that is true most often or circle both. Tally the numbers of your A, B, and C responses below.

Skin

A. Is your skin dry?

B. Is it freckly or prone to redness, breakouts, or rashes?

C. Is it milky, thick, moist, with large pores?

Sleep

A. Do you toss and turn at night, challenged to fall asleep or stay asleep?

B. Do you sleep easily and wake up easily but sometimes rouse around midnight?

C. Do you sleep like a log and enjoy resting in bed in the morning?

Digestive Fire

A. Is your digestion sensitive, with occasional bloating, gas, or constipation?

B. Is your appetite regular and strong, making you fierce if you don't eat?

C. Is your appetite sluggish, especially in the morning, and your metabolism slow?

Thirst

A. Is your thirst variable?

B. Is it strong, sometimes almost insatiable?

C. Do you have low thirst, and do you prefer warm water and teas?

Body Temperature

A. Do your hands and feet run cold?

B. Are you usually warm whatever the season?

C. Are you like a bear, with good insulation but slightly cool to the touch?

Hair

A. Do you have curly, dry, or frizzy hair?

B. Is your hair straight, fine, or fair?

C. Is your hair thick, full, wavy, or oily?

Eyes

A. Are your eyes small, sometimes dry?

B. Do your eyes sometimes get red, itchy, or irritated?

C. Are your eyes large?

Temperament

A. Are you active, quick-witted, curious, engaged, and *sometimes* spaced-out or nervous?

B. Are you competitive, passionate, bold, and *sometimes* impatient or jealous?

C. Are you steady, loyal, forgiving, nurturing, responsible, and *sometimes* melancholic and attached to the past?

Mind

A. Is your mind active, creative, inventive, even intuitive?

B. Are you insightful, clear, focused, determined?

C. Do you have a positive outlook and a strong faith?

Concentration

A. Is your attention quick, short, variable?

B. Is it strong, focused, attentive to detail?

C. Is your focus enduring, mostly expansive, seeing the big picture?

Senses

A. Are you sensitive to sounds? Or to the feel or energy of a place or person?

B. Do you enjoy visual beauty? Do you describe things in full color?

C. Are you the first to notice the aroma of food, flowers, and fragrances?

Self-Identity

A. Do you think of yourself as intellectual, imaginative, spiritual, or inventive?

B. Do you consider yourself to be a motivator, a good coach or leader?

C. Do you value your loyalty to family, friends, alma mater, and hometown?

Mood

A. Does your mood change rapidly?

B. Are you more of a slow burn?

C. Is your mood generally steady?

Under Stress

A. Do you get restless, anxious, worried, or forget to eat?

B. Do you take charge, perspire, break out, or get irritable or impatient?

C. Do you become quiet or pensive, or do you oversleep, overeat, or even become depressed?

Frame

A. Are you light, with a thin frame?

B. Are you athletically built and naturally muscular?

C. Are you curvaceous or well built?

Weight

A. Do you lose weight easily?

B. Does your weight more or less remain steady?

C. Do you gain weight easily, and lose it with difficulty?

Rhythms

A. Do you dislike routine, regularity, and schedules?

B. Does your face flush when embarrassed, or does it flush more often in Summer?

C. Do you get seasonal allergies?

More Signs

A. Do you have joint pain?

B. Is your hair gray, thinning, or bald?

C. Do you experience water retention?

Results ➤

Results

A: VATA

If you chose A for the majority of questions, you are creative, inventive, imaginative, light-footed, and usually lighthearted. You sometimes live in your head, or on the dance floor—in any case, swirling and twirling with ideas and inspiration.

B: PITTA

If you chose B for the majority of questions, you are strong, bold, warm, focused, and determined—the first to the rescue, or to the finish line. Your clarity, courage, and organizational ability make you a great leader and coach, great at uniting people around a powerful vision.

C: KAPHA

If you chose C for the majority of questions, you are kind, patient, protective, family-oriented, and a lover of tradition. Generous with loved ones and quick to offer a helping hand, you are the glue that holds together relationships, families, communities, and healing partnerships.

Balancing These Energies

As a healing science focused on balancing doshas, Ayurveda teaches us that the key is in the application of opposites. For example, heat, as in a spicy tea, a cooked meal, a warm blanket, or a loving touch, helps warm and calm the cold, airy qualities of Vata. Water hydrates the dryness of air, so soups and warm baths are helpful to Vata, and the earthiness of root vegetables grounds the ethereal element of space.

Pitta heat can be cooled by water. Pitta intensity can be relieved by the element of space and is liberated by air. Swimming in the sea, gazing at the night sky, walking through open lands, turning on a fan, or even just observing the flow of each breath—the spaciousness of the inhale, the release of the exhale—are cooling elixirs to balance Pitta.

Kapha is balanced with fire, as in aerobic exercise that makes you sweat, spicy foods that increase the digestive fire, and mental challenges that require focus. Wet, heavy Kapha can also be balanced by the light, dry air element. Strong breathing exercises open the respiratory channels and increase circulation. Circulating out in the world by trying new things, meeting new people, and exploring new ideas brightens and relieves.

Everyone is unique in their expression of the dynamism of the doshas. While there is usually one dosha that dominates, some people have two, and occasionally all three doshas are equivalent.

Doshas	In Balance	Out of Balance
Vata	Strong *Prana* steady energy regular appetite regular elimination	Impaired *Prana* erratic energy irregular appetite gas, constipation
Pitta	Strong *Tejas* steady appetite clear eyes, lustrous skin strong digestion	Impaired *Tejas* sharp hunger red irritated eyes skin eruptions loose stools, bile
Kapha	Strong *Ojas* wakeful energy light in body moderate appetite	Impaired *Ojas* sluggishness, stagnation mucus overeating, indulgence in sweets

If more than one dosha dominates, you could be Vata-Pitta, Pitta-Kapha, Vata-Kapha, or "tri-doshic." When seeking to balance these dual or triple types, people are often confused at first. But there is a simple trick: Consider what the doshas have in common.

Vata-Pitta is both light and mobile, so when imbalanced, earth and water ground and soothe.

Pitta-Kapha contains water. The air element helps both doshas circulate, while space helps them lighten up when they find themselves too singularly focused or weighed down.

Vata-Kapha has both cold and needs a warming touch. Cooked foods and aromatic spices boost the inner fires.

Vata-Pitta-Kapha is like nature itself and just as nature maintains balance through the seasons, Vata-Pitta-Kapha must align with the seasons for optimal balance.

While the doshas describe your imbalances and give an Ayurvedic practitioner insight into the underlying cause of illness, they are *not who you are*. You are a dynamic, complex, and integrated play of *prana*, *tejas*, and *ojas*. With a little understanding and a diet of balanced Ayurvedic recipes, you can feed those inner forces of vitality, radiance, and strength while nourishing your spirit and bringing more creativity into your life.

Appendix A offers more details to help you refine your knowledge and self-awareness. You may also find it helpful to consult someone you trust so you can get a broader view of your overall life tendencies. The doshas are based on simple principles, but we humans are complex and it often takes a qualified Ayurvedic doctor to properly determine your doshic condition.

The Qualities of the Doshas

Everything in nature is perceived through its qualities. Despite the great complexity of nature, Ayurveda identified 20 qualities, also called attributes, expressed as pairs of opposites. Hot or cold, heavy or light, wet or dry, and smooth or rough are some of the most common. For a complete list of these 10 pairs of opposites, see Appendix C.

As with everything in nature, the doshas have their own attributes. According to one of the prime Ayurvedic texts, the *Ashtanga Hridayam*, the qualities of the doshas are as follows:

Dosha	Vata	Pitta	Kapha
Elements	Air + Space	Fire + Water	Water + Earth
Principles	Mobility Connection	Transformation Digestion	Cohesion Structure Lubrication
Function	Catabolic (breaks down)	Metabolic (converts)	Anabolic (constructs)
Qualities	Dry Light Cold Rough Subtle Mobile	Oily/Wet Sharp Hot Light Liquid/Spreading Mobile	Heavy Cold Oily/Wet Smooth Soft Stable/Static

The Qualities of the Seasons

The seasons mark the passage of time over the course of a year and demonstrate how the five elements and their qualities play out dynamically.

Spring is oily/wet, cold, liquid/spreading, and heavy. With its promise of new growth, Spring brings melting snows, rising rivers, often rain or fog, making us feel the weight of Kapha.

Summer is usually warm and often humid. While Summer brings nature in full bloom, Summer is Pitta season, when too much heat can cause depletion and burnout.

Autumn is cold, light, dry, and rough. As days get colder and darker, nature begins conserving energy in this Vata season, when it retracts its life force and scatters golden leaves to the wind.

Winter is cold, dry, and hard. Combining the doshas of Vata and Kapha, Winter is nuanced gray alternating with sharp clear days, and for many it is the season of hard earth, frozen icicles, chapped lips, and chest colds.

Like the doshas, the seasons are dynamic. Springtime may begin heavy, cold, and wet, but Spring moves toward Summer, heating up as it goes. Summer can be hot and moist, but it usually gets cooler and drier in its later months. Autumn is cooling and drying, and these qualities intensify as Winter comes on.

These are general seasonal patterns, of course, and not every climate follows these rhythms. Many areas have less variation in seasons, while others have one season that is long and extreme, like Alaska with its long winter. Wherever you live, you become habituated to the cyclical climate, however dramatic or subtle. Paying attention to the weather in your region and noticing all the ways it affects you enables you to work with Ayurveda to maintain balance and wellness according to your own life's seasons and moods.

Notice the seasons, and allow yourself to observe their qualities. Create rituals to honor each one as it comes. Marking the passage of time with honored festivities helps us accept change with grace and equanimity.

The Qualities of Time

TIME OF DAY AND THE DOSHAS

Even time has doshic intervals, so in any given day there are certain patterns. Early morning is subtle and light; upon waking, our minds are usually clear. At midday the sun is strongest and it's usually the hottest time of day. In the evening, we begin to slow down, and we might start to feel dull or heavy as our bodies prepare to rest for the night. This is the flow of Vata, Pitta, and Kapha throughout the day.

Time of Day	Qualities	Dosha
2:00 a.m.–6:00 a.m. 2:00 p.m.–6:00 p.m.	Light, subtle, cold, clear	Vata
6:00 a.m.–10:00 a.m. 6:00 p.m.–10:00 p.m.	Dense, stable, heavy, dull	Kapha
10:00 a.m.–2:00 p.m. 10:00 p.m.–2:00 a.m.	Sharp, mobile, clear, subtle	Pitta

DOSHAS ACROSS A LIFETIME

As children, we are soft and sweet, and generally prone to colds and heavy mucus, so childhood is said to be the Kapha years. From our teens to the general age of retirement, we are focused on work and numerous responsibilities. These are the Pitta years, when the fire of courage, clarity, and strength is needed. Finally, our later years are marked by the air and space qualities that dry and deplete, but also uplift through travel, hobbies, or spiritual practice. These are the Vata years.

Age	Element/Quality	Dosha
Infant to Teen	Water/soft, smooth, wet, dull	Kapha
Teen to Retirement	Fire/hot, sharp, clear	Pitta
Senior Years	Air/dry, light, cold	Vata

The 20 Qualities and Food

Food is where the play of the 20 attributes (see Appendix C) becomes most tangible—and delicious. Imagine the taste of an olive or celery, an avocado or peanut, an apple or raspberry, and immediately you can probably think of at least one quality that describes it. You might experience the olive as oily, celery as cold or rough, avocado as soft, peanut as hard, apple as watery, and raspberry as light. While all the qualities are considered in designing meals for the doshas, the primary considerations for a healing Ayurvedic meal are *cold or hot* and *heavy or light*. Cold balances Pitta, while hot balances Vata and Kapha. Heavy is harder to digest and will need to be prepared in ways to make it lighter, while light foods may need to be made more grounding for Vata.

Qualities	Foods
Cold versus Hot	cucumber versus ginger
Light versus Heavy	lettuce versus cow's milk
Oily/Wet versus Dry	olives versus rye
Mobile versus Stable	sprouts versus sweet potato
Smooth versus Rough	yogurt versus celery
Subtle versus Gross	saffron versus beef
Sharp versus Dull	chile pepper versus wheat
Soft versus Hard	avocado versus firm cheese
Dense versus Liquid/Spreading	banana versus lemon juice
Clear versus Cloudy/Sticky	ghee versus butter

Practice Perfects

Beyond theory, taking these Ayurvedic concepts into your own direct experience will help you develop a more intimate relationship with the world and with yourself. Ayurveda is asking you to be the scientist, the observer, and the knower. Meditating upon these elements, qualities, and tastes brings alive your own inner guru, and enlivens your own inner healer. This is what I love most about Ayurveda: It is knowable, personal, and affirming.

Chapter 2 goes into greater detail on the 20 qualities as they relate to food and Ayurvedic cooking. You will find related tables and charts in Appendixes A and B.

Guiding Principles in Ayurveda

While it treats each individual as unique, Ayurveda is governed by universal principles. Here are five simple practices to cultivate and sustain optimal wellness, no matter what your dosha.

1. Enjoy Nature

Go for a walk, dig up a garden, or sit by a window on a Winter afternoon and watch the snow fall. Observe the forces of sun, soil, wind, and water, and how they interact. Notice what nature, this living intelligence, does on any given day, in any given moment. Take deep breaths in a forest, let the warmth of the sun kiss your face, root your feet into the earth, and feel the dance of prana, or the essential life force, in and around you.

If you live in an urban environment, go to a park, or find a tree and study it, or at the very least acknowledge nature's insistence on life–the grass growing up through tiny cracks in the cement, or the winged insect who finds an open window and a sweet place to land no matter what the weather. Bring nature indoors with houseplants, herbs for the windowsill, and, of course, fresh fruits and vegetables from the farmers' market.

2. Live by the Seasons

When you live by the seasons, you benefit from nature's healing balance, naturally and with ease, because each season has its own inherent balancing intelligence.

In Summer, the sun gives us warmth, light, and vitality, inspiring us to get out and play. To balance the heat, Summer's bounty is alive with cooling foods such as squash, melons, cucumbers, and a variety of juicy fruits and berries.

Autumn weather is typically windy, dry, and cool. We toss on our sweaters, sip spiced teas, and seek warmth in community or at home by the fire. This is the season of grains and root vegetables that must be cooked and are more flavorful with digestive-enhancing spices, and of fermented foods like krauts and yogurts that keep us warm and grounded while strengthening immune function.

Winter is the season to rest and replenish, to sip steaming hot bowls of soup, and gather around the fire with the comfort of friendship and the inspiration of the new year. Like Autumn, this is the season of grains, roots, and fermented foods, but in these colder, darker, and drier days, we are drawn to make more soups and stews with more pungent spices for warm hydration.

In Spring, snows melt and rivers swell. There can be rain, dew, or fog. To avoid feeling soaked and swollen, we stay warm and dry and delight ourselves with Spring's fresh harvest of stimulating, pungent roots and tubers; drying, astringent vegetables and purifying bitter greens; and the light, bright tang of citrus.

3. Opposites Attract— and Heal

One of the most charming and astute observations of Ayurveda is that *like likes like*. In other words, the doshas like their qualities and perpetuate them. Fire likes heat. Air likes to move. Water seeks low ground.

The principle here is usually described as *like increases like*. It suggests that patterns reinforce themselves, especially once they build momentum. If you've ever found your-

Balancing Energy from Within

Given that all the qualities arise from the space, air, fire, water, and earth elements—which, in turn, arise from the *prana*, *tejas*, and *ojas* forces that are already inside of you—with concentration you can summon balancing energy from within. If you are feeling a quality like heavy, for instance, you can imagine yourself light as a feather. If you feel hot, imagine an ice cube on the back of your neck. If you feel ungrounded, imagine you are a tree with deep roots. Your imagination can be a great healer because the mind is powerful, and the essential qualities are always within.

self laughing and you can't stop, eating ice cream when you are sad, or staying up late at night to finish a project, then you've found yourself inhabiting this principle.

It's an Ayurvedic application of Newton's law of inertia, where energy continues as is, at rest or in motion, unless something interferes. Visualize a ship at sea. Once it revs up its engines and sets itself on course, it seems to move without effort. It's an elegant principle, demonstrating nature's efficiency in conserving energy.

If you like the course the ship is taking, all is well. But what if you want to turn that ship around? To counter its inertia, you need a lot of force. The engines rev at full force as that mighty ship makes a wide turn and gradually builds speed in the opposite direction.

With this practice of achieving balance through the application of opposites, Ayurveda presaged Newton's second law of motion, and his third law, too: To balance or transform a force, an opposing force in equal or greater measure must be applied.

The beautiful thing about nature is that while similar qualities accumulate, opposites attract. Vata people often love Yoga and other embodying practices that ground and center. Pitta people usually love water, berries, and roses. We are naturally attracted to that which balances and restores us. We just have to let our innate wisdom guide us.

Try it now: Notice how you feel. Describe the quality of this sensation to yourself. Think of its opposite. Consider where this opposite quality exists, and apply it. Notice how the application of an opposite quality affects you.

On a day when you feel light, eat a roasted sweet potato for lunch. If you feel your heart hardening, cuddle a soft puppy. If you feel heavy, get up and dance.

It's intuitive, instinctive, and harmonizing. It's when we go against this natural wisdom that we create imbalance; *prajnaparadha* is the Ayurvedic term: disrupting or ignoring our natural intelligence.

Learn to embrace your balancing opposites. Let the mutual attraction grow, and watch how that restores and heals.

4. Cultivate Your Vital Essence

Ayurveda is a science of the life force, teaching us the basic language of life energy and its organic functioning in the body.

The Ayurvedic term *dosha* comes from the Sanskrit root *dush*, meaning "to spoil." Dosha refers to that which darkens, weakens, or causes things to decay. Imbalanced doshas bring about disease.

When in balance, the doshas support *prana*, *tejas*, and *ojas* as the primary forces and subtle substances behind all physiological and psychological functions. In the right relationship, *prana*, *tejas*, and *ojas* create the sweet hum of effortless well-being.

An Ayurvedic tenet is that optimal health is the proper unobstructed flow of *prana* through the channels of the body and mind. We increase *prana* through deep breathing, practicing Yoga, inspired thinking, and positive creative pursuits.

Tejas is inner radiance, the subtle energy of fire, through which we digest impressions and thoughts. It can be cultivated through contemplation, concentration, silence, studying nature, and meditation. In the belly, *tejas* becomes *agni*, the power of fire, to digest, metabolize, and transform. *Agni* is crucial to wellness, so supporting it is essential. This is a subject we explore in greater depth in chapter 2.

Ojas is strengthened with the right diet, proper rest, spiritual practices, devotion, and service to others. Renowned Ayurvedic physician Dr. Vasant Lad describes *ojas* as the end product of digestion, containing all five elements, nourishing the hormonal, reproductive, and autoimmune systems, and giving "intelligence ... spiritual energy and power."

While *tejas* relates to digestion, *prana* is the energy released from the foods properly digested, and *ojas* is the end product of digestion. With digestion such a critical factor in producing good *prana*, *tejas*, and *ojas*, Ayurvedic cooking is a primary tool in healing and promoting vibrant living.

Remember that you are nature, and consider how you reflect the qualities of each element. Be kind, positive, and affirming as you do this. After all, the purpose of Ayurveda is to strengthen the positive.

5. Your Belly Is a Brain

Did you know that your digestive tract has more nerve cells than your entire spinal cord? That every known neurotransmitter in your brain is also present in your gut? That 95 percent of serotonin, a mood-enhancing hormone, is found in your digestive system, instead of your brain? Scientists like Michael Gershon at the Columbia University Medical Center and Emeran Mayer at the UCLA School of Medicine have been making these fascinating discoveries in their work in the field of neuro-gastroenterology, which studies the complex connections between our brain and our gut.

Have you ever had an experience that made you feel sick to your stomach? Or found yourself snacking when you felt restless, even though you were not hungry? Stress alters appetite. So much so that Robert Sapolsky, a Stanford neuroendocrinologist and expert on the effects of stress on human behavior, observed that stress can cause two-thirds of people to overeat and the remaining third to undereat.

Correcting the Imbalances of Doshas

Your health and well-being are determined by the state of your dosha, so knowing your own unique combination of the elements and how to maintain balance will give you greater health and fulfillment in life.

Vata

Vata people have a lot of *prana*, so they are quick moving, quick-witted, quick to learn, and lighthearted. Their inspiration makes life exciting and fun. When Vata is in balance, they feel agile, free, creative, and curious.

When Vata is out of balance, Vata people feel light-headed, accident-prone, and ungrounded. To balance Vata, focus on slowing down, and centering and grounding yourself, while gently spicing and warming your meals, and resting your active mind. Take deep breaths and restore your positive *prana* in nature. Cultivate *tejas* through mantra meditation and *ojas* with deep, consistent rest.

Pitta

Pitta people have good *tejas*, so they are warm, radiant, bold, passionate, and clear. When Pitta is in balance, they are great leaders, coaches, and adventurers. They feel strong, focused, and centered.

When Pitta is out of balance, irritability or inflammation rise up. Take a deep drink of water, go for a swim, exhale to release intensity, laugh to restore lightness, and take breaks to create a sense of spaciousness. Cultivate positive *tejas* by visualizing beauty; *prana* by walking, stretching, or creative play; and *ojas* through forgiveness or service to others.

Kapha

Kapha people exude lustrous *ojas*, making them gentle, grounding, encouraging, and patient. When Kapha is in balance, they are tireless teachers, nurturers, counselors, and caregivers, with an unflagging energy, steady faith, and warm family relations. When Kapha is out of balance, they become sluggish, lethargic, and stuck.

To balance Kapha, crank up the heat with hot spices and exercise. Get active in your community. At home, create space by cleaning out drawers, closets, and the kitchen pantry. Do not hit the "snooze" button, and avoid daytime naps. Cultivate positive *ojas* with right diet, singing and laughing every day, and helping others. Increase *tejas* by getting up at dawn to meditate on the rising sun. Increase *prana* with strong, rhythmic breathing.

Try not to attach yourself to any one dosha but to simply see that, like all things in nature, doshas ebb and flow. We can benefit from their energies, and when they become too much, we can assert mastery with the tools Ayurveda gives us.

For optimal health, remember the mind-body connection: Eat when you are hungry, and eat when you are happy. Otherwise, don't eat. As a rule, Ayurveda recommends we eat in silence, with serenity of heart.

If you do feel tension just before a meal, one of the quickest ways to relieve stress is to engage one or more of your senses. Notice the aromas; savor the flavors. Another way to set the mood for a meal is to remember that nature gives us exactly what we need. Our meal is an offering to our inner fire, to be transformed into energy, intelligence, and strength. For this, we give thanks and bless our food.

While there is an abundance of practices in Ayurveda, here is my quick five for healthy living: eat right, move, rest well, laugh heartily, and forgive.

1. **Eat right:** Choose food that is fresh, seasonal, and balancing for your type.

2. **Move:** Shake it up and move vigorously every day.

3. **Rest well:** Ayurveda finds that the proper amount of rest resolves 80 percent of our problems.

4. **Laugh heartily:** Shake the cobwebs out of your mind and soar free with the power of body-folding, belly-shaking laughter each day.

5. **Forgive:** It heals the heart, restores your loving spirit, and makes room for better things to come.

Ayurveda invites you to a celebration of life itself. The Ayurvedic kitchen is where the feast of that celebration is created—where Mother Nature's colorful harvest serves up delicious plates of *prana*, *tejas*, and *ojas* to nourish you—body, mind, and soul.

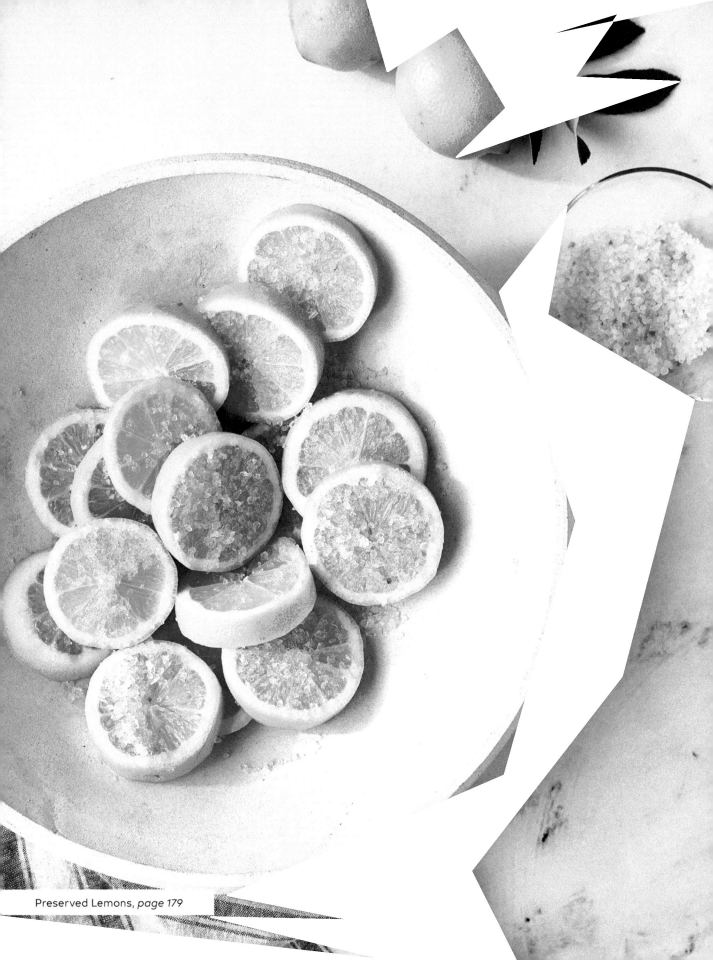

Preserved Lemons, *page 179*

two
Ayurveda & Food

Let food be thy medicine, and medicine be thy food.

–HIPPOCRATES OF KOS, ancient Greek physician

Hippocrates's eternal advice articulates the very essence of Ayurveda. Your body is made up of trillions of cells, each one of which is created and nourished by food. In fact, depending on the source, its preparation, and an individual's capacity to digest it, the same food that supports one person could be harmful for another. In this chapter, we'll take a closer look at foods that balance and heal each dosha.

The Role of Food in Ayurveda

From this very self (atma), did space come into being; from space, air; from air, fire; from fire, the waters; from the waters, earth; from the earth, plants; from plants, food; and from food, human life. Human beings are formed from the essence of food.

—TAITTIRIYA UPANISHAD

Pure, whole foods come from the garden of this Earth we call Mother. Every cell, every tissue, every organ, your eyes, your heart, your kidneys, your stomach, your lungs, your bones and toes—*everything* began as food.

Unlike allopathic medicine, where medicines can be the first line of defense, Ayurveda turns to medicines, usually herbal formulas, only *after* adjusting diet and lifestyle. This honors the body's intelligence while empowering patients to take charge of their own health—and to do it creatively and deliciously in the comfort of their own homes.

You Are What You Digest

Long ago, when people lived more in tune with nature, the wise ones knew intuitively that our digestion is like a fire mirroring the fire of our sun. They could feel on their skin that when the sun is high in the sky, it is warmer, and when it is low in the sky, as it is in the morning and evening, it is cooler, and they understood from this that our digestive capacity must be greatest at midday when the fires are strongest but weaker at sunrise and sunset.

Ever since, traditional peoples have made the midday meal their largest. This is the time of day to enjoy foods that are more difficult to digest: foods that are cold and fibrous like salads and raw vegetables, or foods that are heavy like meat, cheese, grains, or nuts.

Mornings and evenings have traditionally been the time for a lighter meal—something cooked and sweetly spiced like oatmeal, cinnamon toast, or soup—to compensate for the diminished digestive fire.

There is an Ayurvedic saying: "Food is sensory. Digestion is divine." Food is experienced through your five senses. It is feeding you *first* through sensory experience. But food feeds your body through the process of digestion. It is through your digestive fire, what Ayurveda calls *agni*, that food—a plant, grain, flower, nut, or seed—becomes your blood, cells, tissues, organs, and bones.

If you have ever experienced digestive trouble, you can relate immediately to the saying "digestion is divine." But the saying goes beyond that: It is a reference to the source of existence as radiance, light, and fire. It is a reminder that life was first forged in the belly of a star, a fiery furnace in the sky. It is another reminder that we are a part of, and a reflection of, the whole, which is naturally radiant and intelligent.

Ama

"Poison" is a strong word for what Ayurveda calls *ama*, a sticky goo that acts like a toxin and can lead to pain, discomfort, and even disease. But anything that leads to disease is like a poison in the system. *Ama* is translated to mean "improperly digested food." When *ama* accumulates in the tissues, it can cause blockages and malfunction, adding stress to the digestive, immune, and hormonal systems. Signs of *ama* include bad breath, a coated tongue, a lack of appetite, unexplained weight gain, constipation, fatigue, weakened immune function, headaches, mood swings, and even depression.

Ama is created when digestion is low or impaired. To avoid the buildup of *ama*, *agni* needs to be strong and balanced. Fresh, seasonal foods, when Ayurvedically prepared and taken in moderation at the right time of day, help restore digestive strength.

The following food combinations create *ama* and should be avoided:

- Beans + Fruit, cheese, eggs, fish, milk, meat, yogurt
- Eggs + Fruit, melons, beans, cheese, fish, milk, yogurt
- Fruit + Any other food (some cooked combinations are okay)
- Grains + Fruit
- Honey + Ghee, anything boiled or cooked
- Hot drinks + Cheese, fish, meat, starch, yogurt
- Lemon + Cucumbers, milk, tomatoes, yogurt
- Melons + Everything
- Nightshades + Melons, cucumbers, dairy products
- Yogurt + Fruit, cheese, eggs, fish, hot drinks, meat, milk, nightshades
- Milk + Bananas, cherries, melons, sour fruits, yeast bread, Kitchari (see pages 98, 103, 110, and 114), fish, meat, yogurt

To keep it simple:

- Don't mix proteins.
- Consider dairy a protein: Don't mix it with beans, fish, or meat.
- Heavy + Heavy = Heavy, and that means it can tax digestion.
- Fruit is best eaten on its own, unless it's a small amount cooked into a dish.

HOW DO YOU SUPERCHARGE YOUR AGNI?

Imagine the digestive system as a large fire. If you add too much wood, you can overwhelm the fire and extinguish it. If the wood is too wet, too heavy, or too hard, the fire struggles and may dwindle or die. If you add artificial materials, the fire gags with toxic smoke, if it is able to burn at all.

Heavy food, too much food, cold food, cold water, old food, and frozen, canned, or processed food can impair or diminish the bright blaze of your digestive fire.

If you feel heavy, sluggish, and cloudy brained, or if you are experiencing mood swings, then you may have a low-burning digestive fire that has resulted in *ama* in your system.

If you think you need to strengthen your digestive fire, try fasting first to clear any clogging, sticky toxins. You can simply skip dinner one night weekly, or stick to a warm, liquid diet for a day. Sip warm vegetable purées and broths for your three meals.

Drinking lemon and ginger tea throughout the day, and always with your meal, will also increase the digestive fire and help reduce *ama*. It's often recommended that you add ginger to your food when cooking too. Avoid unhealthy food combinations, and try to eat fresh, home-cooked meals as much as possible.

Good Food Combining

Breakfast: a hot bowl of grains, warmed fruit, or a brothy vegetable soup

Lunch: wholesome grains, mung beans, a steamed vegetable, followed by a small glass of warmish buttermilk

Dinner: traditionally a soup, or light stew, or steamed vegetables

Good snacks: fruit, nuts, or seeds, if truly needed

The quality of your *agni* will determine your capacity to digest foods based on their qualities, which is why Ayurveda focuses primarily on the qualities of cold/hot and heavy/light. A weak *agni* will be depleted further by foods that are cooling and/or heavy, while hot and light can encourage good digestion.

The Gunas

Imagine a fruit tree in the Spring. Its branches extend, leaves grow, flowers blossom, and eventually it bears fruit. When that fruit is ripe, you pluck it and take a bite. Its juicy, sweet taste fills you with delight.

But let's imagine you eat only half of the fruit and toss the other half onto your compost pile, where it eventually decomposes back into the soil that will support next year's growth. Ayurveda describes this ever-evolving cycle of life, dissolution, and rebirth as the state of the *gunas*: *Rajas* is the tree growing its fruit, *sattva* is the fruit perfectly ripe, and *tamas* is the fruit decomposing to support the future cycle.

The Gunas and the Mind

Sattva: light, clarity, purity, harmony, balance, creativity, positivity, peace

Rajas: dynamism, passion, stimulation and overstimulation, attachment, aggression, lust

Tamas: darkness, stagnation, heaviness, dullness, decay, dissolution, greed

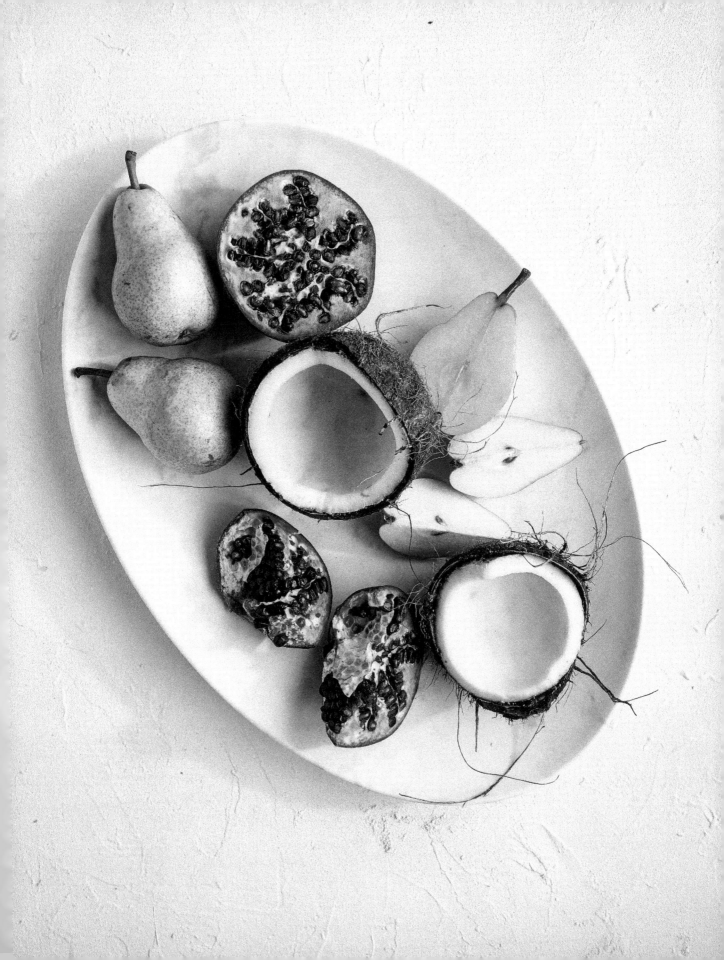

In Ayurveda, the *gunas* are considered especially in terms of the mind. While all things in nature cycle through each of these states, the goal for human development is to reach and maintain *sattva* as much as possible. A *sattvic* mind is loving, clear, truthful, magnanimous, single-pointed, and pure. *Sattva* aids the healing process, and gives the clarity and ease necessary to make the right choices for your best health.

Gunas and Food

Your brain is a hungry organ, consuming roughly 20 percent of your daily calories. Just as the quality of your food determines the quality of your body tissue, the quality of your food feeds the quality of your mind.

Ayurveda describes three basic food groups that correspond to the *gunas* and affect our daily moods, focus, and energy: foods with the energy of goodness (*sattva*), foods with the energy of stimulation (*rajas*), and foods with the energy of dullness and decay (*tamas*).

Sattva: fresh, organic, seasonal, locally grown produce

Rajas: stimulating foods that are spicy, salty, sugary, or fried

Tamas: foods that are canned, frozen, highly processed, stale, or unhealthy when combined (such as fruit and dairy)

For balance, clarity, ease of digestion, lightness in body and mind, good energy, and life vitality, we should eat balancing, light, *sattvic* foods. Which is why in this book we focus on *sattvic* foods such as:

Fruit: Mango, pomegranate, coconut, fig, peach, pear

Vegetables: Sweet potato, lettuce, parsley, cilantro, sprouts, squash

Grains: Rice (especially basmati), quinoa, amaranth

Legumes: Mung beans, lentils

Dairy: Whole milk, buttermilk, paneer, ghee

Sattvic meals include Kitchari (page 98), steamed vegetables, buttermilk, fruits, nuts, and seeds, as an example. The recipes in this book are based on the principles of *sattva*.

The Six Tastes of Food

Nature's evolutionary, self-regulating, and nourishing intelligence is conveyed to us through her foods. Each flavor of nature's bounty expresses a different ray of this intelligence, becoming a powerful tool in crafting a sumptuous, balancing, and satisfying meal.

The Six Tastes

From the five elements, with their 20 qualities, arise six categories of foods based on taste. Each of the six tastes has a vital role to play in our physiology, health, and well-being.

1. **Sweet:** Strengthening, nourishing, tonifying, and satisfying, the sweet taste combines the elements of earth and water. Its qualities are heavy, wet, and cold, and it associates with the emotions of love and bliss, or greed when consumed in excess. Sweet increases Kapha while decreasing Pitta and Vata. It is the primary taste in grains, fruits, root vegetables, nuts and seeds, dairy, eggs, and meat.

2. **Sour**: The sour taste is primarily the result of acids, which are stimulative, digestive, energizing, and moistening. Combining the elements of fire and earth, the qualities of sour are hot and heavy. Sour increases Pitta and Kapha while decreasing Vata. It is the primary taste found in yogurt, cheese, vinegar, and other fermented foods such as miso, pickles, beer, and wine.

3. **Salty**: Soothing and softening, increasing salivation, digestion, absorption, and elimination, salt combines fire and water. With the qualities of hot and wet, salt increases Pitta and Kapha, while decreasing Vata. Seaweed, seafood, sea salts, celery, and cottage cheese express the salty taste.

4. **Pungent**: Improving digestion, absorption, elimination, and circulation, as well as warming the body and clearing the senses, the pungent taste comes from the fire and air elements. With the qualities of hot, light, dry, and pungent, it decreases Kapha while increasing Pitta and, in excess, aggravating Vata. The pungent taste is in peppers, ginger, garlic, onions, leeks, mustard greens, radishes, and turnips, as examples.

5. **Astringent**: Astringency absorbs, contracts, lightens, decongests, helps binds the stool, and inhibits bleeding, sweating, and diarrhea. Combining air and earth, its qualities are dry and cold. The astringent taste decreases Pitta and Kapha while increasing Vata. It is the primary taste in cabbage, apples, pears, persimmons, and the skin of many fruits and vegetables, and it is a secondary taste in legumes and beans.

6. **Bitter**: Detoxifying, purifying, and antibacterial, the bitter taste stimulates the flow of digestive juices and clears stagnation from the blood. The bitter taste is made up of air and space, with the qualities of dry, cold, and light. It decreases Kapha and Pitta while increasing Vata. The bitter taste is in leafy greens, artichokes, eggplant, bitter melons, sesame seeds, coffee, and dark chocolate.

You can enhance flavor in your meals with less salt by stirring in a sunny squeeze of lemon, a spoonful of fermented vegetables like sauerkraut, or a generous garnish of fresh herbs like basil, mint, or dill.

Foods for the Dosha

Vata

When Vata is dominant, focus on the sweet, sour, and salty tastes, with foods that warm, strengthen, and ground.

Include foods that are liquid or unctuous to balance dryness, some heavy foods for grounding and sustained nourishment, foods that are smooth in texture to offset roughness, and foods that are warm or hot to balance the cool nature of Vata.

Fruits, root vegetables, grains, mung beans, seeds, nuts, nut milks, buttermilk, and high-quality fats are ideal for Vata, along with gentle spices like ginger, cinnamon, and nutmeg to optimize digestion. Sipping ginger tea throughout the day will help keep Vata warm and hydrated.

Equally important for Vata is regularity in the timing of your meals. Eat breakfast, lunch, and dinner at the same time each day. Consistency will improve digestion and give you better energy.

Pitta

When Pitta is dominant, focus on the sweet, bitter, and astringent tastes with foods that cool, soothe, and sustain.

Include foods that are cool to balance the fiery quality of Pitta, some heavy foods for enduring sustenance, and a few dry foods to balance the secondary watery nature of this dosha.

Fruits, vegetables, grains, seeds, legumes, and dairy or nut milks are ideal, while ghee is the optimal high-quality fat. Avoid pungent spices, opting instead for cooling herbs like mint, dill, cilantro, and fennel.

For optimal hydration, add lime, cucumber, or mint to your water instead of ice, and sip at regular intervals throughout the day.

Kapha

When Kapha is dominant, focus on the pungent, astringent, and bitter tastes with foods that are light, dry, and stimulating.

Favor foods that are spicy and cooked to balance the cold quality of Kapha, foods that are nourishing but light to counter the heaviness of Kapha, and a few dry foods, like toast or popcorn, to balance the water element in Kapha.

Vegetables, especially leafy greens, citrus and light fruits, lighter grains like quinoa, legumes, and seeds versus nuts, are ideal for Kapha, especially when cooked with strong spices such as ginger, cinnamon, clove, cayenne, mustard, basil, oregano, turmeric, or pepper.

Skipping dinner one night a week helps revive Kapha digestion, and a daily mug of turmeric, ginger, black pepper, and lemon with hot water will stimulate metabolism.

When you include all six tastes in a natural, whole-food meal, all five elements are fed, so your body is fully nourished. Because you are satisfied, your cravings diminish. Most important, you build healthy tissue, increase energy, strengthen the immune system, and boost mental acuity. When you have a meal balanced with all six tastes, you feel nature's intelligence harmonized within you.

The science of the six tastes teaches us that we don't need to count calories or measure protein-carbohydrate-fat ratios. We simply need to savor our way to wellness—remembering that vigorous, vitalized health is never more than six tastes away.

Putting It All Together

Your dosha is the energy predominant in this moment, whether it is due to the weather, the season, your lifestyle and habits, or today's mood. Doshas are balanced by the opposing qualities inherent in each of the six tastes.

Each season has a dosha, which nature balances with foods of opposite qualities. Eating seasonally helps maintain balance and optimal wellness. This is true for everyone, *whatever your personal dosha.*

In the season that corresponds to your dosha, this is especially true, because your tendency to imbalance will be fed by that season's energies, whereas the foods unique to that season will be your key foods for balance.

As an example, Spring is Kapha season, making it a vulnerable time for people with Kapha dosha. While the pungent, astringent, bitter harvest of spring is good for everyone, anyone with a Kapha dosha will especially benefit by adhering to Spring's seasonal bounty and recipes. Likewise, Summer can aggravate Pitta, and Autumn can weaken Vata, but locally grown foods available in these seasons offer balance.

That is why this is the easiest place to start: Eat seasonally and adjust to your dosha.

If you have Vata dosha, you may have to consistently address an irregular digestive fire, so in choosing seasonal ingredients and recipes, favor the sweet, salty, and sour tastes. Lightly cook and gently spice your meals, and minimize cold, drying, and rough foods like salads, raw vegetables, toast, and popcorn.

For Pitta dosha, in every season, favor the sweet, astringent, and bitter tastes. Reduce the salty, sour tastes like yogurt, fermented foods, and alcohol. Minimize spices and include some raw foods with your lunchtime meal.

For Kapha, pursue balance by following the seasons in food choices and preparation while adjusting recipes with hot spices. Favor light, cooked meals and the pungent, astringent, and bitter tastes while decreasing heavy, oily, cold, sweet, salty, and sour.

Ayurveda encourages us to learn about the world through our five senses and to cultivate our own personal relationships with food, doshas, nature, and life itself. The following tables give you an overview, but nothing replaces your own body's wisdom, so explore for yourself your best foods and recipes for each season.

Dosha	Tastes That Increase Dosha	Tastes That Balance Dosha
Vata	Bitter, Astringent, Pungent	Sweet, Salty, Sour
Pitta	Sour, Pungent, Salty	Bitter, Astringent, Sweet
Kapha	Sweet, Salty, Sour	Pungent, Bitter, Astringent

Keeping it simple: Local foods available in each season naturally balance the dosha of that season, so keep life simple with these three rules: seasonal, sattvic, and six. Including foods that are seasonal and locally grown, sourced, and prepared in a sattvic manner, and balanced in the six tastes at every meal, will naturally support your digestion, metabolism, radiance, and intelligence.

Ayurveda teaches us to fully taste the qualities of life and appreciate the variety of flavors in our meals. The joy of this awareness, tasting each experience, is itself a healing, harmonizing practice.

Season	Dosha	Qualities	Tastes to Decrease Dosha
Spring	Kapha	Cool, Heavy, Wet	Pungent, Bitter, Astringent
Summer	Pitta	Hot, Moist, Light	Bitter, Astringent, Sweet
Autumn	Vata	Dry, Light, Cool	Sweet, Salty, Sour
Winter	**Vata-Kapha**	Dry, Heavy, Cool	Sour, Pungent

The recipes in this book take all of this into account, so you can head straight to the recipe section, get into your kitchen, and start cooking. Or, if you are curious to learn more, see Appendixes A and B, and Resources.

Five Ayurvedic Principles for a Healthy Diet

Now that you've got the math—5 elements, 3 doshas, 20 qualities, 3 gunas, and 6 tastes—let's simplify it into a plan with these 5 basic principles:

1. Seek *sattva*.
2. Eat seasonally.
3. Balance all six tastes.
4. Adjust to your dosha.
5. Combine wisely.

If you follow the first rule, you are covered. *Sattvic* foods are light, balancing, and full of *prana*, so they are energizing, intelligent, and nourishing.

Because *sattvic* foods are fresh from nature, they are seasonal—they are what nature is growing for you to balance the dosha of that season. *Sattvic* foods are easy to balance for the six tastes and for your dosha. In fact, when we are healthy, our body naturally craves the foods for the right balance.

When you are in the habit of eating *sattvic* foods, you will notice what food combinations are aggravating because your belly will tell you. Until your feedback loop is fine-tuned enough to always let you know what nourishes you and what doesn't, consult the food combining chart (page 27) to guide you.

Foods to Reduce

Remember, Ayurveda believes that food can be either medicine or poison, depending on the source, the preparation, and the individual's *agni*. For example, raw honey can be medicinal, yet cooked honey is toxic. Chile peppers can mitigate Kapha, but will aggravate Pitta. Any food that impairs your digestion is likely to be ama producing, potentially feeding a chronic imbalance and thus considered "a poison."

Foods that are fried, processed, canned, or frozen, as well as commercial dairy products, baked goods, sugar, and processed meats, can disrupt digestion.

Other foods are natural, and even healing, but can still have *rajasic* or *tamasic* effects on the body, behavior, mind, and consciousness. For example, garlic and onions are said to lead to greed, selfishness, and overindulgence when cooked and eaten in excess, or they can lead to anger and irritation when eaten raw. However, they also can be potent medicinals if used sparingly.

While processed sugar is best avoided, Ayurveda uses a boiled sap of the palm tree or sugar cane called *jaggery*. A cross between molasses and brown sugar, jaggery is considered a particularly good *anupan*, or a medium for delivering medicines, especially in certain conditions of Vata dosha. Used in very small doses, jaggery can balance Vata and slightly decrease Pitta, while not aggravating Kapha. If you can find jaggery, use it whenever sugar is called for in a recipe. Otherwise, coconut sugar is a better choice than refined sugar.

Salt improves your capacity to taste by increasing water on the tongue, and natural salts contain a number of minerals essential for cellular and cognitive function. When using salt, always choose a natural salt. Good salts go by names like pink salt, Himalayan salt, rock salt, mineral salt, and sea salt.

However, salt does increase the water element, so it should be reduced in the case of excess Kapha. It is also a trigger for certain Pitta conditions like hypertension and migraines, in which case it will need to be reduced or even eliminated.

Lemon is a great substitute for salt, spices boost the flavor complexity of a meal, and really fresh ingredients have more flavor naturally, requiring less salt to compensate.

What About Meat?

Ayurveda is the sister science of Yoga. Thus, the first principle of Yoga, *ahimsa*, meaning "first do no harm," is an important principle in Ayurveda, too. With Yoga, the commitment to *ahimsa* assumes a high level of adherence, and many Ayurvedic practitioners are Yogis, who are vegetarians as part of this commitment. However, Sage Charak wrote a chapter on wholesome foods in his seminal Ayurveda textbook the *Charaka Samhita*, listing certain animal meats as nourishing and stating that the "use of meat soup is best in curing emaciation."

Still, those were ancient days when animal husbandry was a more natural, personal enterprise. Nowadays there are so many considerations, and this is a deeply personal choice.

Ayurveda understands that living consciously and compassionately includes caring for your own needs, even as you respect the needs and dignity of others.

If you do choose to include fish or meat in your diet, I invite you to commit to supporting conscious farming methods and compassionately raised animals. Prepare these heavier foods with dosha-appropriate spices to help digestion, and keep at least half of every meal plant-based. That way, you can feel good knowing you are eating according to your values, which will in turn impact your digestion and improve our world.

Cultivating Your Digestive Fire

Given that everything we eat either nourishes or depletes our cells, tissues, organs, and bones, it is essential that we feed our bodies the best-quality nourishment—and that we help our bodies optimally *process* that food.

This is where *agni* comes in. When you eat, you think you are feeding your body. But Ayurveda believes you are feeding your fire. It's that fire that transforms food into a healthy body and mind.

To cultivate your digestive fire, consider implementing these habits:

- Favor warm, cooked foods prepared from fresh ingredients.
- Eat in a calm environment, with attention paid to each taste, and chew thoroughly.
- Sip ginger or mint tea with your meals, avoiding iced or carbonated drinks.
- Consider the wisdom of good food combining: Prepare meals with ingredients that support each other and in their harmony support you.
- Mind the seasons and adjust for your dosha.
- Sip warm water throughout the day.
- Eat only when hungry, and stop when you feel full.

- Be a sun chaser: Eat your largest meal at midday; keep morning and evening meals light.
- Complete digestion before your next meal. Avoid snacking unless you're hungry. Respect your digestive fire: allow it to do the job it's meant to do, and try not to interrupt while it's working. Digestion is complete when your body sends the signal of hunger. Until then, avoid snacking and give each meal the space it deserves.
- Give it a rest: Skip dinner one night a week to allow your inner fires time to catch up.

To restore weakened digestive fires, eat a little ginger before your meals:

- Chop an inch of peeled, fresh ginger into matchsticks. In a small bowl, stir together fresh lemon juice and a pinch of pink salt. Add the ginger sticks and marinate for one hour. Eat one ginger stick 30 minutes before each meal.

Right Makes Might: Healthy Routines

Hitabhuk, Mitabhuk, Ritabhuk: "Who is healthy?" Sage Charak legendarily asked. His student, later the Ayurvedic scholar Vagbhut, replied, "One who eats healthy, eats according to need, and eats according to daily and seasonal rhythms."

Right Quality

Always eat warm and fresh. Look for natural, organic produce grown close to home, by happy people. If organic foods tax your budget, check out "The Dirty Dozen and the Clean Fifteen" on page 203 for a list of what needs to be organic and what doesn't.

This is about right relationship with you—loving yourself enough to give yourself the best.

Right Quantity

Too much food overwhelms digestion, leading to *ama*. But how much is enough? Ayurveda has a saying: "Fill your belly one-third with food, one-third with liquid, one-third with spirit." Eat slowly. If you chew well and pause between bites, you will eventually notice your body signaling that it has had enough.

Put your hands together side by side, palms facing up, as if you are about to receive a pouring of your favorite berries. This is the approximate size a meal should be. Ayurveda calls this one *anjali.* Whatever you can hold in your palms is a good measure for any meal.

Anjali actually means "offering." Don't you love what that implies? As Mahatma Gandhi said, "Nature provides for our need, but not for our greed." We take what we need, bless it, and leave the rest for others to enjoy. This is a way of practicing right relationship with the world.

Right Balance

Include all six tastes to make a dish that is delicious and a meal that is fulfilling. Adjust proportions according to your dosha. It may sound like a lot of food or a lot of effort to get all six tastes in, but it can be as simple as adding a sprinkle of spice or a pinch of lemon zest.

Right balance is about being in right relationship with the dynamism of nature—paying attention to what is happening within you and all around you, and adjusting to the needs of the moment with creative care.

Right Timing

As previously mentioned, our digestive fire is said to mirror the sun. In the morning and evening, the sun's rays are light and cool, while the strongest, hottest rays are at midday. Breakfast and dinner should be lighter meals. Since our fires are cooler in the morning and evening, digestion is usually improved by cooking and lightly spicing these meals.

The common Western breakfast of dry cereal with cold milk and orange juice is unfortunately not ideal. Instead, porridge, pancakes, eggs, or toast ignite healthy digestion. For dinner, salad, leftovers, or frozen microwaved foods are unhelpful. Try substituting soup, curry, or stir-fry for warm comfort.

If time is an issue for you, soups and stews can be made ahead and warmed up before serving in the evening. But don't avoid it—preparing your meals is one of the quickest and deepest ways to restore right rhythm to your daily life. Cultivate a relationship with your food, and cooking will quickly go from a chore to a sonata in the symphony of life.

This is being in right relationship with time. It helps master the progression of life, maintaining grace and equanimity through the rhythms, seasons, and years. Many Ayurvedic professionals consider regularity of the right meals to be the most important of these steps, arguably more important even than the quality or quantity of food, because of the way it affects digestion.

Right Mind

All life is a relationship with the world. You are alive because of the life that came before and the life that surrounds and sustains. You belong to this world. You are alive on purpose. You are an integral part of the whole.

Cultivating the practices of the right relationship at every meal not only encourages good health and better energy, it grows self-respect and expands your feelings of interconnectedness.

So try to always eat in a pleasant environment in a peaceful frame of mind. Avoid noisy places or activities like watching television or listening to loud and abrasive music. Feed all five senses by listening, looking, touching, smelling, and tasting with quiet attention. Offer a prayer of thanksgiving and a smile to those who brought your meal from the earth to the table.

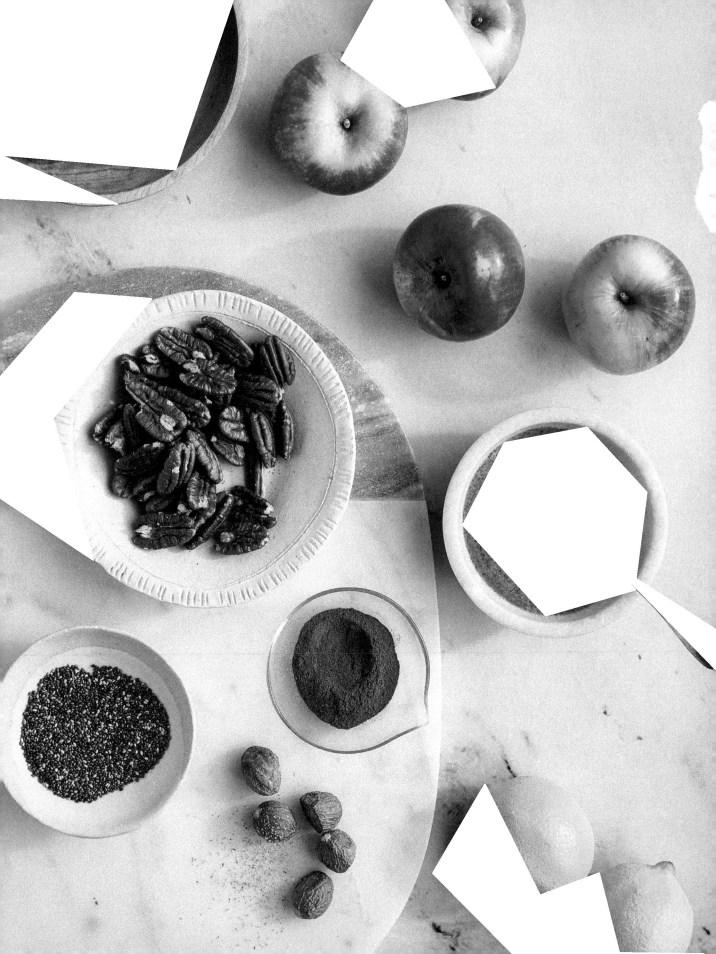

three
Five Steps to
Ayurvedic Eating

Let food be your first medicine and the kitchen your first pharmacy.

–TAITTIRIYA UPANISHAD

The kitchen was once the *hearth*, the heart of a home, where food was cooked and family gathered for warmth and merriment.

Whether your kitchen is large or small, professional or simple, Ayurveda suggests that your kitchen should be like the heart— red, pulsing, and full of love.

The color *red* stimulates digestion. Consider adding a painting, a vase of flowers, or a central visual piece that is red to invoke fire power. *Pulsing* because a kitchen should be a hub of buzzing life— a creative space full of living foods where you can share vibrant joy with family and friends while you cook.

Love because as the poet Rimbaud wrote, "The sun, the hearth of affection and life, pours burning love on the delighted earth." The kitchen is the hearth where we pour burning love into our meals.

Five-Step Plan Introduction

I think of Ayurveda as a science of biophysics, in a language we can understand, with scientific observations we can make ourselves, with our own five senses. Ayurveda looks at patterns, energy, and flow. It's a dance of the doshas, a dynamic interaction of the five elements.

As a science, Ayurveda seeks to create positive flow by establishing new habits and building a powerful momentum.

One way to ensure success is to build incrementally. Pick one new thing this week—pick the most exciting, or the most important, thing—and make a plan to build your week around that one new thing.

Next week, add another new thing. Continue adding one new thing each week. Before you know it, you will have established a pattern of Ayurvedic cooking, as well as establishing expertise in the kitchen, and a way of living that encourages optimal flow.

Here is an outline to get you started.

Step 1: Examine Your Doshic Environment

It is a fact of the brain that it is easier to see and recognize what is around us than to perceive and interpret what is within. This is why we see the greatness of others yet often don't see our own, and it's one reason it can be difficult to assess our own doshic makeup. Another reason it can be difficult is that we are a *dynamic* interplay of all doshas—constantly shifting, changing, balancing, and rebalancing—and it's hard to pin down something that is always moving.

As you explore the elements at play in your own nature, why not invite friends to participate? You can organize a gathering to compare doshas, and lovingly help each other identify individual strengths of *prana*, *tejas*, and *ojas*, with a discussion of the climate where you live and the doshic nature of the seasons. You can also share ideas for incorporating balance, and then support one another in taking new steps and building momentum.

It may seem like a lot to learn and incorporate, but it is simply a question of noticing one thing: How you are feeling today? As Socrates said, "Wisdom begins with wonder."

Follow these three simple steps, and you will benefit from Ayurvedic kitchen wisdom: Eat seasonally, eat *sattvically*, and adjust for your dosha by enjoying foods and spices that are specifically balancing for you. "The Three Doshas" on page 10 is a good guide to begin discovering your doshic tendencies, and Appendix A allows you to explore in more depth.

Did you know that spices can have up to 50 times the antioxidants of fruit? Spices can help heal and protect the gut. Experiment with dosha-appropriate spices to boost the flavor and the medicinal value of your meals.

Step 2: Plan Your Meals

I am often asked how to make a meal for a group of people with varying doshas. How to balance everyone's differing needs? The answer is easier than you might think.

First, any meal that includes all six tastes is balancing to all doshas. Unless someone is very imbalanced, a six-taste meal is enough. Second, in the case of any imbalance, keep meals simple, light, fresh, and easy to digest. This will suit all doshas. Third, prepare a large single-course meal and adjust portion size and spicing for individual doshas.

For example, say you make rice, mung dal, and sautéed greens for a group. A person with Vata imbalance can make the rice their largest portion, and add an extra dollop of ghee or stir in their favorite warming spice. A Pitta can have equal portions and add a generous garnish of fresh cilantro, mint, or dill. A Kapha can reduce the portion of rice, favoring instead the dal and the greens, and sprinkle with red pepper flakes.

Below are four seasonal seven-day meal plans. To really follow these plans would require a lot of cooking, more than most people do day-to-day. So use the meal plans as templates, and be creative. Repeat days that work well for you. Cook leftovers from lunch into a soup for dinner. Pick one day of the week to prepare foods in advance. To turn simple meals into a song, keep your kitchen stocked with some of the basics—spreads and sauces, like the Hot & Spicy Oil (page 64) or Sweet & Spicy Oil (page 65), Preserved Lemons (page 179), or Cilantro Pesto (page 174).

Start where your deepest need lies: what to do for breakfast, how to make healthy dinners, or how to fire up digestion, as examples. Or follow your greatest curiosity: exploring what Ayurvedic rhythms are best for daily meals, how to adjust recipes for the doshas, or what spices support you through the seasons.

Seasonal Seven-Day Meal Plans

Spring Meal Plan

Breakfast: Amaranth Chai Porridge (page 87)

Lunch: Spinach Paneer (page 100)

Dinner: Asian Noodle Soup (page 130)

TUESDAY

Breakfast: Easy Homemade Jam (page 171) with toast

Lunch: Spring Kitchari (page 98)

Dinner: Restorative Roots & Shoots Broth (page 121)

WEDNESDAY

Breakfast: Seasonal Fruit Compote (page 89)

Lunch: Kerala Cauliflower Stew (page 117)

Dinner: Mung Bean Soup (page 120)

THURSDAY

Breakfast: Breakfast Soup (page 91)

Lunch: Beans & Greens (page 101)

Dinner: Ginger Broccolini (page 125)

FRIDAY

Breakfast: Creamy Quinoa (page 86)

Lunch: Tofu Tamari Bowl (page 108)

Dinner: Simple Saag (page 124)

SATURDAY

Breakfast: Buckwheat Pancakes (page 94)

Lunch: Delicious Dal (page 115)

Dinner: Miso Soup with Asparagus (page 122)

SUNDAY

Breakfast: Breakfast Crêpes with Cinnamon-Orange Honey (page 92)

Lunch: Asparagus & Barley Bowl (page 99)

Dinner: Creamy Watercress Soup (page 123)

Summer Meal Plan

MONDAY

Breakfast: Coconut-Mango Crumble (page 169)

Lunch: PLT Sandwiches (page 156)

Dinner: Mung Bean Soup (page 120)

TUESDAY

Breakfast: Creamy Quinoa (page 86)

Lunch: Persian Cucumber Salad (page 105)

Dinner: Curried Green Beans (page 135)

WEDNESDAY

Breakfast: Easy Homemade Jam (page 171) with toast

Lunch: Beans & Greens (page 101)

Dinner: Summer Gazpacho (page 127)

THURSDAY

Breakfast: Breakfast Chia Pudding (page 90)

Lunch: Tofu Tamari Bowl (page 108)

Dinner: Sweet Potato Jackets (page 157)

FRIDAY

Breakfast: Peaches & Cream Smoothie (page 79)

Lunch: Summer Kitchari (page 103)

Dinner: Flatbread Pizza (page 151)

SATURDAY

Breakfast: Rice Pudding (page 84)

Lunch: Mango & Cabbage Salad (page 106)

Dinner: Cauli Tacos (page 149)

SUNDAY

Breakfast: Buckwheat Pancakes (page 94)

Lunch: Berry & Peach Panzanella (page 104)

Dinner: Mint Pea Soup (page 126)

Autumn Meal Plan

MONDAY

Breakfast: Rice Pudding (page 84)

Lunch: Tofu Tamari Bowl (page 108)

Dinner: Chapatis (page 69) and Avocado Mash (page 184)

TUESDAY

Breakfast: Seasonal Fruit Compote (page 89)

Lunch: Pistachio Rice with Tahini Yogurt (page 113)

Dinner: Roasted Roots Ecrasse (page 129)

WEDNESDAY

Breakfast: Crunchy Yogurt Bowl (page 88)

Lunch: Sesame Noodle Stir-Fry (page 111)

Dinner: Ginger–Carrot Soup (page 131)

THURSDAY

Breakfast: Nutty Oatmeal (page 85)

Lunch: Kerala Cauliflower Stew (page 117)

Dinner: Restorative Roots & Shoots Broth (page 121)

FRIDAY

Breakfast: Breakfast Soup (page 91)

Lunch: Autumn Kitchari (page 110)

Dinner: Sweet Potato Jackets (page 157)

SATURDAY

Breakfast: Nutty-Crusted Apple Pie (page 166)

Lunch: Roasted Vegetable Bowl (page 109)

Dinner: Rice Biryani (page 132)

SUNDAY

Breakfast: Coconut & Mango Crumble (page 169)

Lunch: Delicious Dal (page 115)

Dinner: Miso Soup with Asparagus (page 122)

Winter Meal Plan

Breakfast: Amaranth Chai Porridge (page 87)

Lunch: Beans & Greens (page 101)

Dinner: Yam Fries (page 150)

TUESDAY

Breakfast: Crunchy Yogurt Bowl (page 88)

Lunch: Winter Risotto (page 116)

Dinner: Curried Green Beans (page 135)

WEDNESDAY

Breakfast: Easy Homemade Jam (page 171) with toast

Lunch: Kerala Cauliflower Stew (page 117)

Dinner: Asian Noodle Soup (page 130)

THURSDAY

Breakfast: Nutty Oatmeal (page 85)

Lunch: Roasted Vegetable Bowl (page 109)

Dinner: Lentil Lasagna (page 146)

FRIDAY

Breakfast: Seasonal Fruit Compote (page 89)

Lunch: Thai Noodle Salad (page 107)

Dinner: Simple Saag (page 124)

SATURDAY

Breakfast: Breakfast Soup (page 91)

Lunch: Winter Kitchari (page 114)

Dinner: Cauli Tacos (page 149)

SUNDAY

Breakfast: Whole-Skillet Hash Browns (page 154)

Lunch: Kitchari "Burgers" (page 144)

Dinner: Healing Kanji (page 141)

Step 3: Shop

PANTRY

- Whole mung beans
- Split mung beans, also called yellow dal or moong dal
- Basmati rice
- Ghee, or grass-fed unsalted butter to make your own (page 58)
- Extra-virgin olive oil
- Coconut oil
- Apple cider vinegar
- Tamari (a Japanese variety of soy sauce that is gluten-free and preservative-free)
- Almonds, cashews, pumpkin seeds, sunflower seeds
- Shredded coconut
- Cocoa powder
- Raw honey
- Maple syrup
- Jaggery or Sucanat

FRESH PRODUCE

- Lemons, limes, citrus, in season
- Apples, berries, seasonal fruits
- Root vegetables, like carrots, sweet potatoes, turnips, according to season
- Leafy greens, in season
- Seasonal favorites like avocado, broccoli, pumpkin
- Fresh peas and green beans
- Fresh cilantro, parsley, other herbs

SPICES/HERBS

- Spring: Ground ginger, cinnamon, turmeric, black pepper, cayenne, or red pepper flakes
- Summer: Ground coriander, turmeric, fennel seeds, mint, dill
- Autumn: Ground ginger, cinnamon, cardamom, whole nutmeg, fenugreek
- Winter: Ground ginger, cinnamon, cloves, turmeric, fenugreek
- General: Mustard seeds (brown), pink or sea salt, whole peppercorns

MISCELLANEOUS

- Whole-milk plain yogurt
- Dates

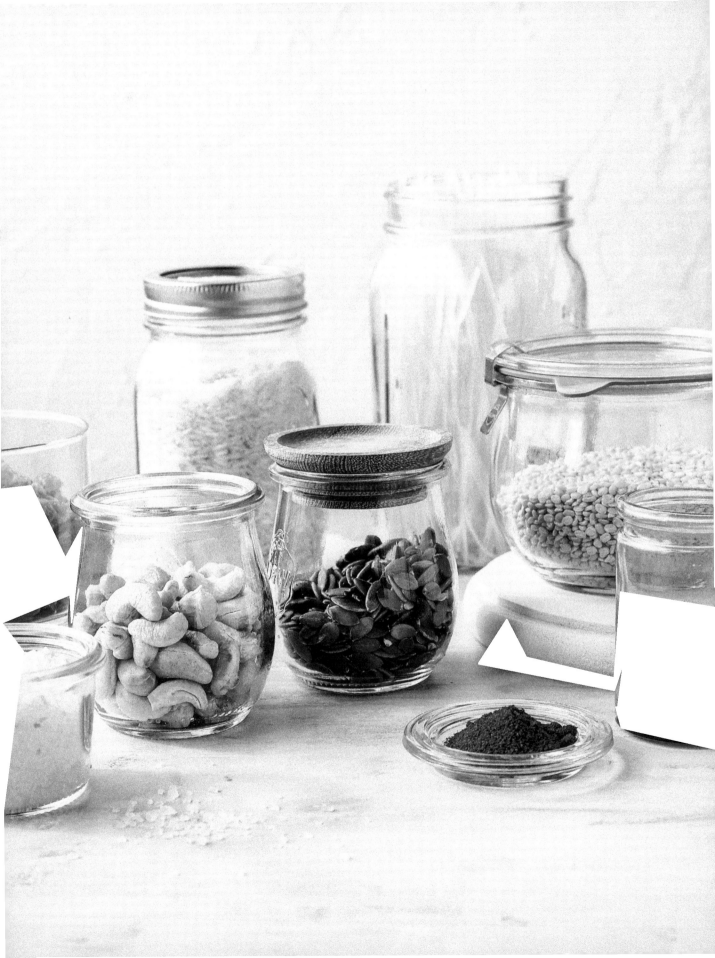

Drink Ayurvedic Teas

So much of Ayurvedic medicine is dispensed in teas. In Ayurvedic clinics, herbs are ground and boiled, sometimes stirred for hours or fermented for months, and often combined in synergistic blends. These herbs transform into a hot and steamy mug of nature's medicine—a nectar to be sipped warm to bring comfort to your spirit and pour through your veins as rivers of healing.

While trained doctors and technicians labor intensively to prepare traditional medicinal teas, there are quick and simple ways to get many of the same benefits at home in your own kitchen.

There are two digestive teas that every Ayurvedic kitchen should include. The first is the Ginger, Lemon & Honey Tea (page 72). This tea is so immune boosting, cold busting, and purifying for the respiratory tract that it is an important first line of defense when seasonal colds loom, and it is excellent for children.

The second tea is the CCF Digest Tea (page 73). *CCF* stands for cumin, coriander, and fennel, which combine to make an all-dosha-balancing tea that is nourishing while cleansing, grounding but light, and warming even as it reduces the internal heat of Pitta.

Step 4: Set Up Your Kitchen

The most essential kitchen tool is a knife. One sharp knife to chop and slice, and another for paring (and a sharpener for both) make a real difference in meal prep. If there is one investment to make, this is it.

In addition to a favorite soup pot and saucepan, I often use a blender, and a box grater for shredding sweet potatoes and carrots. A lemon squeezer is a great help, and a citrus zester will encourage you to add healthy zest to more of your meals.

Mason jars are excellent for storing nut milks, sauces, and really anything, and they are essential for making fermented foods, like the Carrot Pickle on page 185.

An electric spice grinder will help with spice blends, although there is almost nothing more Ayurvedic than grinding by hand, for which a mortar and pestle offer better control and muscular rewards.

I like to always have cheesecloth available for making ghee, and empty paper tea bags to fill with spice blends I want to share. I use glass measuring cups to determine ingredient amounts when baking. Otherwise, amounts are determined by a pinch of the fingers, a scoop of the hands, a seasoned eye, and a lot of tasting.

Ayurveda recommends using hands, fingers, sight, sound, smell, and taste as a way of developing your feel for the kitchen. Trust, empower, and liberate your creative juices by using measuring tools less, your five senses and intuition more. See what comes from cooking by your own perfect measure.

Step 5: Cook with Love and Awareness

In her book *The Path of Practice: A Woman's Book of Ayurvedic Healing*, Bri Maya Tiwari relates the story of a woman who sent a care package to her father, a political prisoner detained a hemisphere away. As she mixed, baked, wrapped, and mailed his favorite treat, she sang the songs of her childhood. In his thank-you letter, her father wrote that he could hear her singing as he unwrapped the package, and felt her love in every bite.

Adding zesty, warming spices to your meals is like adding natural fuel to your fire. By encouraging healthy *agni*, improving the bioavailability of nutrients, and increasing the rate of digestion, spices help leave you feeling light and bright after meals.

In Italy, respect for even the best, most sophisticated restaurants is eclipsed by the respect for mamma's kitchen. Mamma's is always best, they say, because she cooks with love!

In India, there is a saying that the best medicine is in your mother's cooking, and that even the comfort food of your childhood can be healing when it reminds you of the love of family.

Every time I have taken a cooking class in Italy or India, whether it is a *nonna* (grandmother) in her home kitchen or a three-star chef in a stainless steel restaurant kitchen, the demonstration always ends with an empathic lesson: Ultimately, it is the love in your hands, they will say, that makes the dish delicious. They declare that love can be tasted, and that it is the most wholesome, healing ingredient of all.

part two | Recipes to Balance & Heal

Ayurveda invites us to taste our way to health. In these recipes you will find a spectrum of flavors, colors, textures, and aromas to beckon you and your loved ones into a sumptuous relationship with food at every meal.

The recipes are clearly organized according to the meal and type—breakfast, lunch, dinner, sweet treats, plus tonics and teas, sauces and spreads—and appear in seasonal order in each chapter.

To keep it simple and help you get started, most of the recipes use only five or fewer main ingredients—not counting ghee, spices, or seasoning. Seasonal spice blends optimize the healing potential of meals while keeping recipes uncomplicated. The recipes also include tips to allow you to customize for each of the doshas.

Each recipe has icons and labels to help you quickly identify what you are looking for.

YEAR-ROUND RECIPES feature foods you can make anytime with a helpful tip to customize the recipe to your taste and changing needs.

SPRING RECIPES feature light, dry, simple foods and pungent, bitter, astringent tastes to balance the heavy, cool, damp qualities of Spring.

SUMMER RECIPES feature light, simple, cooling foods that focus on the sweet, bitter, astringent tastes to balance the hot, moist qualities of Summer.

AUTUMN RECIPES feature warm, simple, grounding foods with the sweet, salty, sour tastes that balance the cool, dry, windy qualities of Autumn.

WINTER RECIPES feature light, simple, warm foods with the sweet, bitter, astringent tastes to balance the cold of Winter.

ONE POT These recipes can be made in one pot on the stove.

30 MINUTES OR LESS These recipes can be prepared, cooked, and served in 30 minutes or less—including a number of recipes that can be prepared in 15 minutes or less.

KITCHEN REMEDY These recipes offer particularly powerful healing benefits and ingredients, such as *lassi*, a yogurt-based drink that supports your digestive fire and immune system, and *kanji*, a rice soup good for an upset stomach or debilitation.

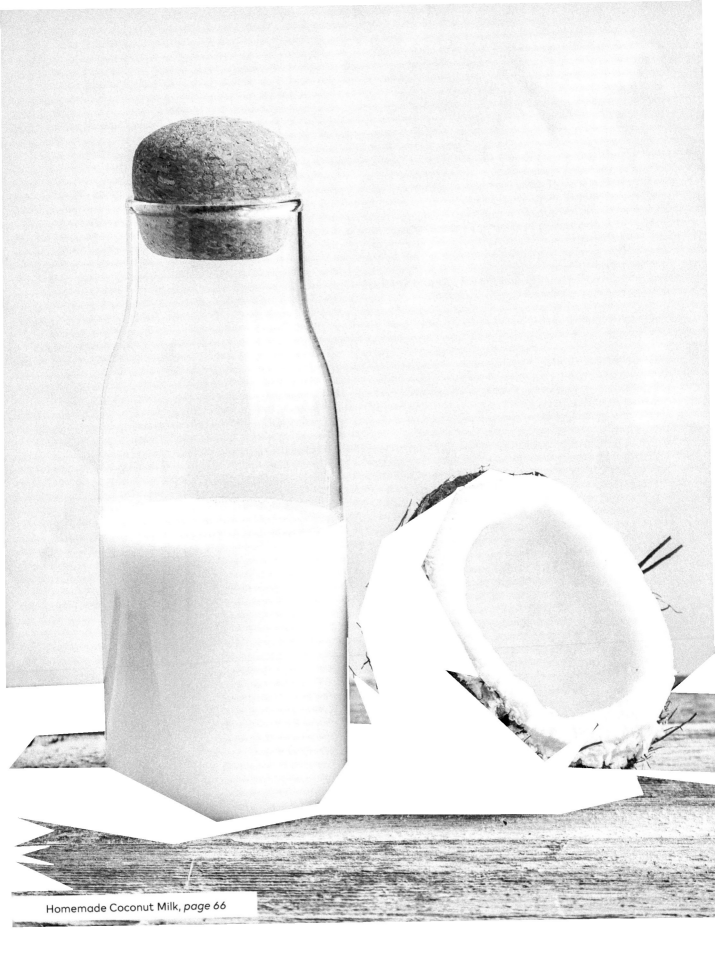

Homemade Coconut Milk, *page 66*

four
Staples & Spices

Ghee 58

Basic Broth 59

Spring Spice Blend 60

Summer Spice Blend 61

Autumn Spice Blend 62

Winter Spice Blend 63

Hot & Spicy Oil 64

Sweet & Spicy Oil 65

Homemade Coconut Milk 66

Homemade Almond Milk 67

Homemade Pumpkin
Seed Milk 68

Chapatis 69

Ghee

One of the most important foods in Ayurvedic cooking is ghee. Preparing ghee is a simple process of clarifying butter by cooking off the casein proteins and fat solids to produce a healthy fat. Ghee helps cultivate *ojas*, the underlying power of immunity and rejuvenation, while delivering unique enzymes that stimulate your digestive power.

MAKES 1 TO 2 CUPS

Prep time: 10 minutes

Cook time: 15 minutes

1 pound pure unsalted butter

1. Melt the butter in a medium saucepan over medium heat. Bring to a boil, then reduce the heat to medium-low.

2. The ghee will foam and gurgle as it releases steam. Once it goes quiet, reduce the heat to low. With a wooden spoon, being careful not to stir the butter, gently push the foam away from the top of the butter. If the butter is transparent to the bottom, the ghee is done. Otherwise, let it cook another minute or two.

3. Line a fine-mesh strainer with cheesecloth. Pour the ghee through the strainer into a clean glass jar. Discard the cheesecloth. Allow the ghee to cool, and secure the jar with an airtight lid.

Storage tip Keep unrefrigerated in a tightly sealed glass jar. Always use a clean utensil. Ghee will keep indefinitely as long as it doesn't become contaminated.

Season Year-round

Dosha All, especially Pitta; use moderately for Kapha.

Basic Broth

ONE POT

Homemade broth has a golden-rich taste you will never find in a store-bought version. Delicious sipped warm from a mug, this broth is the flavor-enhancing foundation for soups, stews, and all the warm bowls that are so plentiful in Ayurvedic cooking.

MAKES 3 TO 4 CUPS

Prep time: 5 minutes

Cook time: 2 hours

1 tablespoon Ghee (page 58)

1 tablespoon Seasonal Spice Blend (pages 60–63)

1 large onion, chopped

4 or 5 large carrots, chopped

1 bunch celery, chopped

4 cups water

1 tablespoon shoyu

1. Melt the ghee in a large soup pot over medium heat. Stir in the spice blend and sauté for 1 minute.

2. Add the onion, carrots, celery, and water. Increase the heat and bring to a boil.

3. Cover the pot, reduce the heat to low, and cook for 2 hours. Turn off the heat.

4. Once the broth cools, stir in the shoyu.

5. Strain and pour the broth into mason jars with airtight lids. Keep in the refrigerator for up to 5 days.

>>> **Cooking tip** As long as you have onion, carrot, and celery as a base, you can add any additional vegetables you like—kale, chard, beets, or whatever is in season. If you aren't feeling well, add chopped ginger or even a few garlic cloves.

Season Year-round

Dosha All

Spring Spice Blend

30 MINUTES OR LESS • KITCHEN REMEDY

Spring spices turn up the heat to help melt the Winter freeze. Stimulating digestive fire, boosting circulation, encouraging the inner channels to open and run clear, these spices make Spring cooking sizzle. This blend goes especially well with soups and as a seasoning for vegetables.

MAKES ¼ CUP

Prep time: 5 minutes

2 tablespoons ground ginger

1 tablespoon
ground cinnamon

2 teaspoons ground turmeric

½ teaspoon cayenne or red pepper flakes

½ teaspoon freshly ground black pepper

1. Put all the spices in a glass jar. Cover tightly with a lid and give it a good shake.

2. Keep in a cool, dry place close to where you cook so it's handy when you need it.

⋙ **Kitchen Remedy tip** Spices are most flavorful and most medicinal when they are fresh. Whenever possible, purchase spices whole and grind them yourself at home. Look for freshly ground spices in your grocer's bulk section, where you can buy only what you need.

🌸 **Season** Spring

🔻 **Dosha** Kapha

Summer Spice Blend

30 MINUTES OR LESS · KITCHEN REMEDY

Summer calls for a cooler approach to cooking, even while the digestive fires still need stoking. This spice blend increases Summer flavor while reducing any accrued heat from the season.

MAKES ¼ CUP

Prep time: 5 minutes

Cook time: 3 minutes

2 tablespoons coriander seeds

2 teaspoons fennel seeds

1 teaspoon dried mint

2 teaspoons dried dill

1 teaspoon ground turmeric

1. Toast the coriander and fennel seeds in a dry pan over medium heat until they are just fragrant and very lightly golden. Remove from the heat and let cool.

2. Put the toasted seeds in a mortar and pestle or spice grinder with the mint, and grind into a fine powder.

3. Pour into a glass jar. Add the dill and turmeric. Cover tightly with a lid and shake to blend.

4. Store in a cool, dry place.

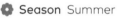 **Kitchen Remedy tip** For a Pitta-reducing Summer refresher, put 1 teaspoon of the spice blend in a pint jar filled with purified water. Add the petals of a rose, a few slices of cucumber, and fresh mint leaves, and let sit in the morning sunlight for a few hours. Strain and enjoy at room temperature with a wedge of lime.

Season Summer

Dosha Pitta

Autumn Spice Blend

30 MINUTES OR LESS • KITCHEN REMEDY

Typically associated with sweet treats, Autumn spices add a rich, earthy tone to seasonal meals, gently easing digestion, warming the body, and comforting the heart.

MAKES ¼ CUP

Prep time: 5 minutes

1 tablespoon
ground ginger

1 tablespoon
ground fenugreek

1 tablespoon
ground cinnamon

2 teaspoons
ground cardamom

1 teaspoon freshly
grated nutmeg

1. Put the ginger, fenugreek, cinnamon, cardamom, and nutmeg in a glass jar, cover tightly with a lid, and shake to blend.

2. Store in a cool, dry place.

⟫ **Substitution tip** Fenugreek is a heavenly spice with a sweet-bitter taste and a soothing, hydrating action on the tissues. It is available online through some of the specialty shops listed in the Resources (page 204). It can be substituted with cumin, which is a great digestive spice but has a strong flavor that not everyone appreciates.

❋ **Season** Autumn

◉ **Dosha** Vata

Winter Spice Blend

30 MINUTES OR LESS · KITCHEN REMEDY

Just as we enjoy stoking the Winter fires, this Winter blend helps stoke the inner fires. With ginger, cinnamon, and cloves, this blend has an aroma and flavors that may remind you of Winter holiday feasts, bringing festive joy to dishes.

MAKES ¼ CUP

Prep time: 5 minutes

2 tablespoons ground ginger

1 tablespoon ground cinnamon

1 teaspoon ground cloves

1 teaspoon ground turmeric

1 teaspoon ground fenugreek

1. Put the ginger, cinnamon, cloves, turmeric, and fenugreek in a glass jar, cover tightly with a lid, and shake to blend.

2. Store in a cool, dry place.

Substitution tip This blend gives a stronger heat than the Autumn blend. It is balanced for Vata and Kapha types, but Vata types may prefer the Autumn blend—in every season. Pitta types may also prefer the Autumn blend and can always use the Summer Spice Blend year-round.

Season Winter

Dosha Vata, Kapha

Hot & Spicy Oil

With its snap, crackle, and pop, this spicy oil is a joy to prepare. It gives you an easy way to modify recipes to an individual dosha by simply stirring a drizzle of spicy oil into the dish after it's been served. It is also a quick way to fire up a sauté, stew, or stir-fry: Just pour in the oil, toss in your fresh ingredients, heat, and serve.

MAKES ABOUT 1 CUP

Prep time: 5 minutes

Cook time: 5 minutes

1 cup Ghee (page 58) or sunflower oil

2 tablespoons brown mustard seeds

1 tablespoon cumin seeds

1 tablespoon ground ginger

1 tablespoon ground turmeric

1. Put the ghee in a pan over medium heat. Add 2 or 3 mustard seeds while it heats.

2. When the mustard seeds begin to pop, remove the pan from the heat. Add the remaining mustard seeds and cover the pan.

3. When the seeds stop popping, add the cumin seeds, ginger, and turmeric. Give the pan a swirl to incorporate the spices.

4. Allow the oil to cool for 5 minutes, then pour it into a glass jar. Cover tightly with a lid and store at room temperature.

⟫ **Substitution tip** Despite its name, this oil is not too fiery. Still, if your digestion is sensitive or you are Pitta constitution, try the Sweet & Spicy Oil (page 65) instead. Stored away from light and heat, this will keep for a few weeks.

✿ **Season** Autumn, Winter, Spring

🜂 **Dosha** Vata, Kapha

Sweet & Spicy Oil

ONE POT • 30 MINUTES OR LESS

A swirl of sweet and cooling spices, this oil enhances flavor without causing you to breathe fire. As with the Hot & Spicy Oil (page 64), you can easily adapt a prepared meal to individual needs by simply drizzling this oil over a dish once it's been served.

MAKES ABOUT 1 CUP

Prep time: 5 minutes
Cook time: 5 minutes

1 cup Ghee (page 58) or sunflower oil

2 tablespoons brown mustard seeds

1 tablespoon fennel seeds

1 tablespoon ground turmeric

1 teaspoon ground cardamom

1. Put the ghee in a pan over medium heat. Add 2 or 3 mustard seeds while it melts.

2. When the mustard seeds begin to pop, remove the pan from the heat. Add the remaining mustard seeds and cover the pan.

3. When the seeds stop popping, add the fennel seeds, turmeric, and cardamom. Give the pan a swirl to incorporate the spices.

4. Allow the oil to cool for 5 minutes, then pour it into a thick glass jar. Cover tightly with a lid and store at room temperature.

➢➢ **Storage tip** Stored out of the light and away from heat, the oil will keep for a few weeks.

✿ **Season** Summer, Autumn

◭ **Dosha** Pitta, Vata

Homemade Coconut Milk

30 MINUTES OR LESS

In Ayurveda, coconut milk is often added to sautés and soups to make a creamy Vata-pacifying, Pitta-balancing sauce. It can also be added to teas, tonics, and smoothies. In the southern Indian state of Kerala, where they are surrounded by coconut trees, many chefs make their coconut milk using this easy method.

MAKES 2 CUPS
Prep time: 5 minutes

2 cups hot water

1 cup shredded coconut

1 teaspoon coconut oil

1. Pour the water over the coconut in a blender. Add the coconut oil and blend on high for several minutes.

2. Lift the lid and scrape down the sides of the blender. Blend for another 1 or 2 minutes, until the mixture is thick and creamy.

3. Pour into a strainer placed over a bowl.

4. Use immediately, or store in an airtight mason jar in the refrigerator for up to 1 week. (The coconut fiber can be blended into smoothies or stirred into a hot breakfast bowl. Otherwise, compost.)

⋙ **Preparation tip** To make a coconut milk for drinking rather than cooking, stir in ½ teaspoon maple syrup, a pinch cardamom, and dash of pink salt after straining.

✿ **Season** Summer, Autumn, Winter, and anytime a dairy alternative is needed.

❂ **Dosha** Coconut milk is creamy, hydrating, sweet, and balancing for Vata. It is sweet, soothing, and cooling for Pitta. Coconut milk is less heavy than dairy, so if thinned and warmed with an additional 1 cup of hot water and a dash of cinnamon, it is a good alternative "milk" for Kapha.

Homemade Almond Milk

Ayurveda loves milk. After all, Ayurveda is a medical practice from India, where the cow is revered. Still, not everyone loves cow's milk or can stomach it, and with the dairy industry being what it is, many people are looking for alternatives. Almond milk is a creamy, nutritious, and delicious choice.

MAKES ABOUT 2 CUPS

Prep time: 5 minutes, plus 8 hours to soak

1 cup raw almonds

2 cups water, plus additional for soaking

2 dates, pitted

1 teaspoon ground cinnamon

½ teaspoon vanilla extract

Pinch pink salt

1. Place the almonds in a bowl and cover with water. Soak the almonds for 8 hours.

2. Drain and rinse the almonds, then transfer them to a high-speed blender along with 2 cups of water. Blend on the highest speed.

3. When the almonds are fully liquefied, pour the liquid through a nut bag into a bowl. Squeeze the bag to release all the milk. Discard the solids.

4. Pour the filtered almond milk back into the blender and add the dates, cinnamon, vanilla, and salt. Blend well.

5. Use immediately, or store in an airtight mason jar in the refrigerator for 4 to 5 days.

>>> **Substitution tip** For Summer, stir in cardamom instead of cinnamon. For Pitta, add rose water and fresh mint for a *sattvic*, cooling tonic.

✿ **Season** Summer, Autumn

❀ **Dosha** Vata, Pitta

Homemade Pumpkin Seed Milk

Pumpkin seeds have a sweet, nutty, and slightly astringent taste. Lighter than almonds, they make a good alternative milk for Pitta and are ideal for Kapha. It's a singular flavor, made sweetly refreshing with the addition of honey, cinnamon, and vanilla.

MAKES ABOUT 2 CUPS

Prep time: 5 minutes, plus 6 hours to soak

1 cup raw pumpkin seeds

2 cups water, plus additional for soaking

1 teaspoon honey

1 teaspoon vanilla extract

1 teaspoon ground cinnamon

Dash pink salt

1. Place the pumpkin seeds in a bowl and cover with water. Soak the seeds for 6 hours or overnight.

2. Drain and rinse the pumpkin seeds and transfer them to a high-speed blender along with 2 cups of water. Blend on the highest speed.

3. Once the seeds are liquefied, pour the milk through a fine-mesh stainless steel strainer into a bowl or pitcher. Discard the solids.

4. Pour the filtered milk back into the blender and add the honey, vanilla, cinnamon, and salt. Blend well.

5. Use immediately, or store in an airtight mason jar in the refrigerator for 4 to 5 days.

>>> **Ingredient tip** Purchase raw seeds in bulk for a better price. (Look for high turnover in the bins for the best freshness and quality.) Or scoop seeds out of a pumpkin and dehydrate them in the sun or in an oven set to a low temperature. Store the seeds in glass jars and keep in a dark, dry place.

✿ **Season** Spring, Summer

△ **Dosha** Kapha, Pitta

Chapatis

From Myra Levin's blog at Hale Pule Ayurveda, I finally got the courage to make chapatis, a thin pancake-like bread of unleavened whole-grain flour cooked on a griddle in just minutes. By making many "mistakes," I learned that you can't go wrong. If you undercook one, pop the chapati back on the griddle. Overcooked, it gets crisp like a cracker. The heat and timing equation will vary, so look for air bubbles when cooking. When the dough stops bubbling, that is the time to flip. Use a whole-wheat or gluten-free baking flour for the best results.

SERVES 2

Prep time: 15 minutes

Cook time: 10 minutes per chapati

1 cup whole-wheat or gluten-free flour, plus 1 tablespoon, for rolling

Hearty pinch Seasonal Spice Blend (pages 60–63)

½ teaspoon salt (pink, mineral, or sea)

½ cup water

1 teaspoon Ghee (page 58), plus additional for cooking

1. Combine 1 cup of flour, the spice blend, and salt in a medium bowl.

2. Mix in the water and the ghee until completely blended.

3. Sprinkle the remaining 1 tablespoon of flour on a flat surface, and roll a handful of dough in your hands to make a ball. Set the ball of dough on the edge of the floured surface and repeat until all the dough is in balls.

4. Add more flour to the surface if needed, and flatten one ball of dough with your hand. Flip to keep it from sticking to the surface, and continue to pat the dough until it is almost as thin as a pancake.

5. Melt the ghee on a griddle or skillet on medium heat. When the ghee is very hot, place the flattened dough on the hot griddle. Cook for about 3 minutes, flip, and cook for another 3 minutes. The chapati is done once it has bubbled and those bubbles are lightly brown on each side.

6. Remove to a plate and cover with a towel while you repeat steps 4 and 5 for the remaining dough.

>>> **Serving tip** Serve alongside dals and soups, or simply with ghee, or with the avocado mash for a rich and nourishing delight.

Season Year-round

Dosha All

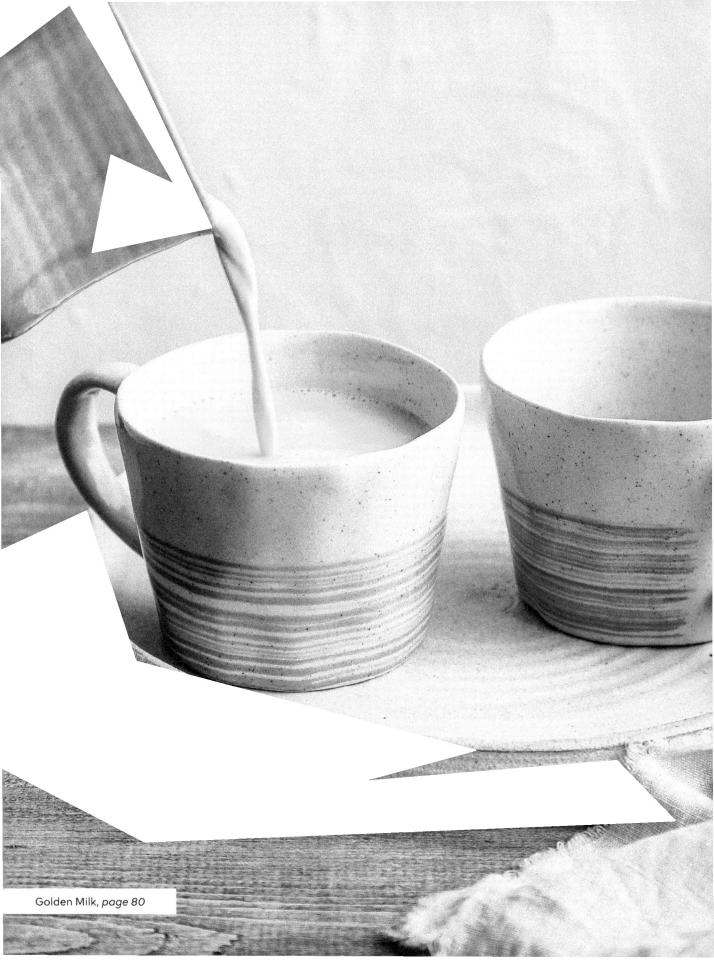

Golden Milk, *page 80*

five
Teas & Tonics

Ginger, Lemon & Honey Tea 72

CCF Digest Tea 73

Coconut Chai 74

Digestive Lassi 75

Rose Lassi 76

Rose Fennel Tea 77

Cucumber-Mint Cooler 78

Peaches & Cream Smoothie 79

Golden Milk 80

Deep-Sleep Tonic 81

Ginger, Lemon & Honey Tea

30 MINUTES OR LESS • KITCHEN REMEDY

Pungent, sour, sweet, and warm, this tea is as medicinal as it is comforting. When I travel, I pack my ginger, lemons, and honey, and ask for hot water everywhere I go—on the plane, in the train, at the hotel, in the cafés. To keep your immune system strong, drink daily in Winter and Spring. To counter a cold, sip throughout the day.

SERVES 2

Prep time: 5 minutes

Cook time: 15 minutes

1 (1-inch) piece fresh ginger

4 cups water

Juice of 1 lemon

2 tablespoons raw honey

1. Peel and chop the ginger into chunks and put in a pot with the water. Cover and bring to a boil, then reduce the heat to low and simmer for 10 minutes. Turn off the heat and steep for another 5 minutes.

2. Once the tea has cooled enough to sip, stir in the lemon juice. Strain the tea and discard the ginger chunks.

3. Ladle yourself a cup of tea. Stir in 1 tablespoon of honey per serving.

⇢⟩⟩ **Ingredient tip** Ginger is known for its capacity to warm, heal, nurture, and restore. Fresh ginger is hotter than powdered ginger, so if you are a Pitta type or if it is Summer, ground ginger is a better choice. If you don't have fresh ginger but want the same strength, stir ½ teaspoon ground ginger into warm water until you get the heat you seek.

❀ **Season** Winter, Spring

🝆 **Dosha** Kapha. For Vata, substitute jaggery or coconut sugar for honey.

CCF Digest Tea

30 MINUTES OR LESS • KITCHEN REMEDY

CCF is short for cumin, coriander, and fennel, the three ingredients in this Ayurvedic staple. CCF Tea aids in digestion, assimilation, metabolism, and purification. Cumin is heating, making it an ideal spice for Vata. Coriander improves digestion while balancing Pitta. Fennel is sweetly pacifying to both Vata and Pitta and lends a delicious licorice-like richness to the taste. Spices are always good for Kapha types who benefit greatly from drinking their liquids hot. This is an all-season tea that, when sipped at regular intervals throughout the day, helps balance the doshas, improve *agni*, and stimulate detoxification. If you're on the go, take your hot CCF with you in a thermos. In Summer, allow it to cool, and serve it with a few leaves of fresh mint.

SERVES 4

Prep time: 5 minutes
Cook time: 15 minutes

¼ teaspoon cumin seeds
½ teaspoon coriander seeds
½ teaspoon fennel seeds
6 cups water

1. Put the cumin seeds, coriander seeds, fennel seeds, and water together in a large pot. Bring to a boil, then reduce the heat to low, cover, and simmer for 10 minutes.

2. Strain the tea and discard the seeds. Pour the tea into a thermos and sip it throughout the day.

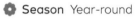 **Substitution tip** Cumin seeds have a strong earthy flavor that some people love while others don't. If you are a cumin lover, you can even increase the amount to ½ teaspoon so all the seeds are equal in amount. If you are not so fond of cumin, try substituting cardamom pods.

✿ **Season** Year-round

◬ **Dosha** All

Coconut Chai

Chai simply means "tea," and it can be made in a variety of ways. When it's brewed with ginger and cardamom, it is referred to in India as *masala chai*. In this version, it's really more of a masala milk with warm, soothing spices that make it a perfect afternoon delight.

SERVES 2

Cook time: 5 minutes

2 cups Homemade Coconut Milk (page 66)

2 teaspoons Autumn Spice Blend (page 62)

½ teaspoon ground ginger

½ teaspoon ground cardamom

½ cup water (optional)

1. In a saucepan, bring the coconut milk, spice blend, ginger, and cardamom to a gentle boil.

2. If you'd like a thinner consistency, whisk in the water and return to a boil. Strain, discard the solids, and serve.

➤➤ **Substitution tip** Almond milk works equally well. For Kapha, use equal parts of water and milk.

⬡ **Season** Autumn, Winter, Spring

◑ **Dosha** Vata, Kapha. For Pitta, use the Summer Spice Blend (page 61) and half the ginger, and allow to cool before drinking.

Digestive Lassi

30 MINUTES OR LESS · **KITCHEN REMEDY**

Your belly will thank you when you finish your meal with lassi, a yogurt-based drink that keeps your digestive fires blazing and your immune system strong. Coconut or rice yogurt substitute well for dairy.

SERVES 2

Prep time: 5 minutes

1 cup whole-milk yogurt

1 teaspoon raw honey

1 teaspoon vanilla extract

Pinch ground cinnamon

Pinch freshly grated nutmeg

Pinch ground cloves

Dash pink salt

Dash freshly ground black pepper

1 cup water

1. Put the yogurt, honey, vanilla, cinnamon, nutmeg, cloves, salt, pepper, and water in a blender and blend until frothy.

2. Enjoy after lunch as a digestive treat.

Remedy tip Equal parts of yogurt and water plus ½ teaspoon fresh grated nutmeg can be restorative to the gut in case of loose stools or diarrhea.

Season Autumn, Winter

Dosha Vata

Rose Lassi

When I am in the desert, I make a very watery version of this and sip it throughout the day to keep hydrated and to fuel the digestive fires. You can find rose water at most grocers, often in the Asian or Middle Eastern section—or you can make it yourself by pouring hot water over a handful of rose petals and allowing it to steep for an hour before straining.

SERVES 2

Prep time: 5 minutes

1 cup whole-milk yogurt

½ cup rose water

1 teaspoon maple syrup

1 teaspoon Ghee (page 58) or coconut oil

Hearty pinch ground cardamom

½ cup water

Pink salt, for seasoning

1. In a blender, blend the yogurt, rose water, maple syrup, ghee, and cardamom with the water until frothy.

2. Taste, adjust the seasoning, add pink salt if needed, and serve.

Substitution tip Substitute dairy yogurt with coconut yogurt. You can also use jaggery or coconut sugar in place of the maple syrup.

Season Autumn, Winter

Dosha Vata. Pitta if digestion is weak.

Rose Fennel Tea

30 MINUTES OR LESS • KITCHEN REMEDY

When life gets hot, busy, or intense, taking a moment to stop and smell the roses can change everything, which speaks to the power of rose to cool, calm, and soothe. This tea is the *sattvic* equivalent of enjoying a healing pause in nature. The ingredients are simple: rose, fennel, and mint. Rose is soothing and astringent. Fennel is a sweet, cooling digestive. Mint is light and refreshing. Together they create a gentle medicine to balance Summer's heat with a delicate, subtle taste that makes you want to slow down and smell, sip, taste, and breathe in the beauty of life.

SERVES 2

Prep time: 5 minutes
Cook time: 10 minutes

2 cups water
1 teaspoon fennel seeds
5 or 6 mint leaves
2 tablespoons rose water

1. Bring the water to a boil in a saucepan.

2. Add the fennel seeds, cover, and reduce the heat to low. Simmer for 3 minutes, then turn off the heat. Allow the seeds to steep for 5 minutes more.

3. Stir in the mint leaves and rose water. Pour through a tea strainer, and serve.

⟩⟩⟩ **Serving tip** You can make this ahead of time and serve it at room temperature, or add cool coconut milk to make an Ayurveda version of iced tea.

✿ **Season** Summer, Autumn

◭ **Dosha** Pitta, Vata

Cucumber-Mint Cooler

30 MINUTES OR LESS • KITCHEN REMEDY

Full of electrolytes and other temperature-regulating minerals, cucumbers are Summer's cooling gift and a useful ingredient for rehydration. Mint is the most cooling herb for Pitta, though it is pacifying for all doshas and excellent for digestion. Lime is a bitter citrus, and the bitter taste combines space and air. This is the refreshment equivalent of opening a window when it is stifling hot to let in a cool, welcome breeze.

SERVES 2

Prep time: 5 minutes

1 medium Persian cucumber, chopped into 3 or 4 pieces

Juice of 1 lime

6 mint leaves, plus additional leaves for garnish

Pinch pink salt

1 cup water

1. Add the cucumber, lime juice, mint, salt, and water to a blender. Blend on high until completely puréed.

2. Pour into glasses, garnish with an additional mint leaf or two, and serve.

Ingredient tip Persian cucumbers have the best flavor with fewer and smaller seeds. They also allow you to use the whole cucumber, including the skin, which has additional nutrients. If you can find only the larger, waxy cucumbers, remove the peel and the seeds before blending.

❀ **Season** Summer

❀ **Dosha** Pitta

Peaches & Cream Smoothie

30 MINUTES OR LESS · KITCHEN REMEDY

For centuries, South Asian cuisine has combined turmeric with coconut milk, which science now shows improves the bioavailability of turmeric, making it more effective in addressing inflammation, cognitive function, cell repair, skin health, and liver health. With basil for a digestive-enhancing flavor boost, it makes an easy Summer breakfast or sweet afternoon refresher. It could even be gently heated for an evening soup, or poured warm over rice.

SERVES 2

Prep time: 5 minutes

1 cup Homemade Coconut Milk (page 66)

2 peaches, pitted

1 apple, cored and quartered

Handful fresh basil, plus additional for garnish

1 teaspoon ground turmeric

Ground cardamom for garnish

1. Place the coconut milk, peaches, apple, basil, and turmeric in a high-speed blender and blend until smooth.

2. Serve with a garnish of basil and a sprinkle of cardamom.

⫸ **Remedy tip** Ice dampens the digestive fire and is therefore avoided in Ayurveda. Add 1 to 2 tablespoons of coconut oil to enhance the turmeric's brain-boosting, joint-soothing, and muscle-smoothing powers.

✿ **Season** Summer

◈ **Dosha** Cooling for Pitta people who can substitute basil for mint. For Vata, blend until it begins to heat up from the friction of the blender, and drink warm. For Kapha, add freshly ground black pepper when blending.

Golden Milk

Turmeric is said to balance all doshas, and research shows it to be cleansing to the blood and lymphatic system, helping dissolve tumors and blood clots, improving circulation, promoting healthy menstruation, healing soft-tissue injury, and decongesting the liver. It also aids in the digestion of sugar, fats, and oils, making it beneficial to those with diabetes and hypoglycemia. Coconut milk is a great substitute for dairy.

SERVES 2

Prep time: 5 minutes

Cook time: 5 minutes

2 cups whole milk

1 tablespoon ground turmeric

Pinch freshly ground black pepper

Small pinch ground cardamom

1. Place the milk, turmeric, pepper, and cardamom in a saucepan. Whisk gently while bringing the milk to a low boil. Remove the pan from the heat.

2. Serve and drink warm.

≫≫ **Ingredient tip** Turmeric has been used to dye fabrics bright yellow. Unless you want sunny patches of yellow on your clothing, wear an apron and handle with care.

Seasons Year-round

Doshas All. Vata people can stir in jaggery or coconut sugar. Pitta people can stir in 1 teaspoon of maple syrup, if needed. Kapha people should dilute with 1 cup of water and stir with generous shakes of ground ginger or cinnamon.

Deep-Sleep Tonic

KITCHEN REMEDY

Ojas is the Ayurvedic word for deep nourishment, our underlying reserves of energy. It is said to derive from wholesome, well-digested foods and rejuvenating rest. Foods that support *ojas* are ghee, nuts, dates, raisins, and milk. If you could use a little help sleeping, try this Ojas-building sleep tonic. Resoundingly popular and potent, it is great for calming Vata, or any flighty, fractured, anxious, can't-settle-down sort of energy. Enjoy it an hour before bed for a night of sweet dreams and deep slumber.

SERVES 2

Prep time: 5 minutes, plus 8 hours to soak

Cook time: 3 minutes

10 almonds

1 cup whole milk

1 teaspoon Ghee (page 58)

3 or 4 dates, pitted

½ teaspoon ground cinnamon

½ teaspoon ground cardamom

½ teaspoon grated nutmeg

Pinch freshly ground black pepper

Pinch ground turmeric

½ cup water

1. Put the almonds in a bowl and cover with water. Soak for 8 hours.

2. Drain and rinse the soaked almonds.

3. Put the almonds, milk, ghee, dates, cinnamon, cardamom, nutmeg, pepper, turmeric, and water in a blender and blend on high speed until the almonds and dates are liquefied, 1 to 2 minutes.

4. Pour the mixture into a saucepan and bring to a gentle boil. Remove the pan from the heat.

5. Pour the tonic into mugs and drink warm.

⋙ **Substitution tip** Replace the almonds with 1 cup of Homemade Almond Milk (page 67) for a quick and easy tonic, or use 2 cups of almond milk to replace both the almonds and the dairy. Be sure the nutmeg is freshly grated, and double the amount if you want increased sleep-enhancing benefits.

⚙ **Seasons** Year-round

◢ **Doshas** Vata, Pitta

Breakfast Crêpes with Cinnamon-Orange Honey, *page 92*

six
Breakfasts

Rice Pudding 84

Nutty Oatmeal 85

Creamy Quinoa 86

Amaranth Chai Porridge 87

Crunchy Yogurt Bowl 88

Seasonal Fruit Compote 89

Breakfast Chia Pudding 90

Breakfast Soup 91

Breakfast Crêpes with
Cinnamon-Orange Honey 92

Buckwheat Pancakes 94

Pumpkin Nut Bread 95

Rice Pudding

ONE POT

A bowl of cooked grains, sweetly spiced, is one of the traditional staples of Ayurveda, and a comforting way to wake up. Fortifying all constitutions in any season, this simple recipe comes together in minutes, and then heats on the stove while you prepare for your day, making it a great way to start any morning, all year round.

SERVES 2

Prep time: 5 minutes

Cook time: 35 minutes

½ cup basmati rice

1 tablespoon Ghee (page 58)

¼ teaspoon ground cardamom

Pinch salt (pink, mineral, or sea)

1 cup boiling water

1 cup Homemade Almond Milk (page 67)

4 dates, pitted and chopped

½ cup golden raisins

1. Rinse the rice in a strainer for a couple of minutes to wash off much of the starch that makes rice sticky.

2. Melt the ghee in a saucepan over medium heat. Add the cardamom and sauté for 1 minute. Stir in the rice and salt, and stir to coat the grains thoroughly.

3. Slowly add the water and stir. Bring to a boil.

4. Slowly stir in the almond milk, maintaining a low boil. Stir, cover the pan, and reduce the heat to medium-low. After 20 minutes, stir in the dates and raisins. Reduce the heat to low, cover the pan, and cook for another 10 minutes. Serve warm with your favorite toppings.

⇉ **Remedy tip** To lighten this pudding, cook with water only, increasing the amount to 4 cups and omitting the dried fruit. Strain, and keep the rice water to sip as a broth.

✿ **Season** Summer, Autumn, Winter

◆ **Dosha** Great for Vata people, who can stir in nuts such as pecans or walnuts, sesame seeds, or fruits such as banana or berries. Good for Pitta people, who can also add berries. For Kapha people, boil the rice with water only and omit the dates.

Nutty Oatmeal

30 MINUTES OR LESS

Oats are a light and digestible grain, yet cook up into a hearty and filling breakfast. This creamy bowl of oats gets a nutty crunch from toasted pecans and pumpkin seeds. Cook with fresh fruit—banana for Vata, berries for Pitta, and apple for Kapha—for doshic-balancing sweetness.

SERVES 2

Prep time: 5 minutes

Cook time: 20 minutes

1 cup rolled oats

2 cups water

1 tablespoon Ghee (page 58)

2 handfuls pecans

2 handfuls pumpkin seeds

1 teaspoon Seasonal Spice Blend (pages 60–63)

1. In a medium pot, bring the oats and water to a boil. Reduce the heat to a simmer and cook for 15 minutes.

2. In a shallow pan, melt the ghee over medium-high heat. Add the pecans and pumpkin seeds and toast them for 1 minute, shaking the pan a time or two to turn the nuts and seeds. Remove the pan from the heat.

3. Ladle the oatmeal into two bowls. Divide the toasted nuts and seeds over the top of the oats.

↠ **Serving tip** Delicious with a spoonful of ghee, a drizzle of maple syrup or honey, or a dollop of yogurt.

✿ **Seasons** Autumn, Winter

◮ **Doshas** Excellent for Vata. For Pitta, reduce the pecans by half or omit them; stir fresh berries into the oats in the last 5 minutes of cooking.

Creamy Quinoa

ONE POT · 30 MINUTES OR LESS

Quinoa makes a light, nutritious breakfast. Delicate and fluffy, quinoa has an astringent quality that pairs well with the sweet of the coconut. Flaxseed enhances the nutty flavor while boosting brainpower to start your day sharp.

SERVES 2

Prep time: 5 minutes
Cook time: 25 minutes

1 cup cooked quinoa

1 tablespoon Ghee (page 58)

1 teaspoon Seasonal Spice Blend (pages 60–63)

1 cup water

1 cup Homemade Coconut Milk (page 66)

½ teaspoon salt (pink, mineral, or sea)

1 tablespoon unsweetened shredded coconut

1 tablespoon flaxseed

1. Rinse the quinoa in a mesh strainer for about 2 minutes.

2. Melt the ghee in a pot over medium heat. Add the rinsed quinoa and toast it for 1 minute, stirring or swirling the pan a time or two. Stir in the spice blend.

3. Pour in the water, coconut milk, and salt. Bring to a boil.

4. Reduce the heat to low and stir in the shredded coconut and flaxseed. Cover and cook for 15 minutes.

5. Turn off the heat and let the pot stand, covered, for 5 minutes. Remove the lid and fluff the quinoa gently with a fork. Serve.

Ingredient tip Quinoa can be bitter or even soapy tasting, but you can make it sweet and nutty just by giving it a good rinse before cooking. Massage the seeds as you rinse, to get to every grain.

Seasons Winter, Spring, Summer. In Spring, replace the coconut milk with Homemade Pumpkin Seed Milk (page 68).

Doshas Pitta. For Kapha, use Homemade Pumpkin Seed Milk in place of the coconut milk.

Amaranth Chai Porridge

ONE POT • 30 MINUTES OR LESS

Paired with Autumn spices and cooked in almond milk, amaranth becomes a warm bowl of sweet comfort. Flaxseed promotes elimination, while the spices enhance *agni*, making this a hearty, nutritious breakfast to fire up a chilly day.

SERVES 2

Prep time: 5 minutes

Cook time: 25 minutes

1 tablespoon Ghee (page 58)

1 teaspoon Autumn Spice Blend (page 62)

½ teaspoon ground cloves

Pinch salt (pink, mineral, or sea)

1 cup amaranth

2 cups Homemade Almond Milk (page 67)

1 apple, cored and chopped

1 teaspoon flaxseed

1. Melt the ghee in a pot over medium-high heat and stir in the spice blend, cloves, and salt.

2. Stir in the amaranth, almond milk, apple, and flaxseed, and bring the mixture to a boil.

3. Reduce the heat to low. Cover the pot and simmer for up to 20 minutes, until the amaranth is fluffy and the water is absorbed.

Ingredient tip Amaranth is a high-protein, gluten-free, ancient grain with a subtle nutty taste. Its light and purifying qualities make it a good rice replacement with any meal.

Season Autumn, Winter, Spring

Dosha For Vata, add more ghee and a drizzle of maple syrup to balance the drying nature of the amaranth. For Kapha, replace the almond milk with water or Homemade Pumpkin Seed Milk (page 68).

Crunchy Yogurt Bowl

Ayurveda loves warm, spiced grains for breakfast. Yet sometimes we want hearty and healthy without having to light up the stove. Quick and easy to make, this crunchy yogurt delivers tasty nutrition when you don't have the time to cook.

SERVES 2

Prep time: 5 minutes

2 cups plain yogurt

2 tablespoons pumpkin seeds

2 tablespoons sunflower seeds

2 teaspoons ground flaxseed

½ cup Homemade Coconut Milk (page 66)

1 teaspoon Autumn Spice Blend (page 62)

1. Spoon 1 cup of yogurt into each of two bowls. Sprinkle the pumpkin seeds, sunflower seeds, and flaxseed over the top of the yogurt.

2. Pour the coconut milk around the rim of the yogurt in each bowl and sprinkle with the spice blend.

>>> **Serving tip** For extra creaminess, stir in a spoonful of Pumpkin Seed Butter (page 181). If you prefer your breakfast a bit sweeter, drizzle in 1 teaspoon of honey.

⚙ **Season** Autumn

◬ **Dosha** For Vata, stir in 1 teaspoon of maple syrup or coconut sugar.

Seasonal Fruit Compote

30 MINUTES OR LESS

Although this recipe is perfect for all seasons, I especially love making it with Winter fruits. In the Winter, dried fruits like cranberries, cherries, and apricots cook up with red apples and orange to create jewels of elegant warmth. Dried fruits swell and glisten with the fruit juices and ghee, suggesting Mother Earth is a queen and fruits are her gems. Stir this into a bowl of breakfast grains, spoon it over toast, or eat it straight up for an afternoon pick-me-up.

SERVES 2

Prep time: 5 minutes

Cook time: 10 minutes

2 apples

1 pear

1 orange, peeled

1 tablespoon Ghee (page 58)

1 heaping teaspoon Seasonal Spice Blend (pages 60–63)

2 cups seasonal berries or dried fruits

½ cup water

1. Core the apples and pear, and roughly chop.

2. Slice the orange into half moons.

3. Melt the ghee in a saucepan over medium heat. Stir in the spices and sauté for 1 minute. Add the apples, pear, orange, and berries, and swirl to coat.

4. Add the water and bring to a boil. Reduce the heat to low, stir, cover the pan, and simmer for 5 minutes. Serve warm.

➢➢ **Remedy tip** When your digestive fire is low, fruit compote is easy on the system, with spices that help reset and restore.

✿ **Season** Year-round

✿ **Dosha** All, especially with seasonal fruits and seasonal, or dosha-appropriate, spices

Breakfast Chia Pudding

This pudding is a refreshing welcome on warm Summer mornings. It's delicious on its own but can also be heated with cooked apples, toasted pumpkin seeds, or your favorite seasonal fruits. The key is to prepare it the evening before, letting the chia seeds stand overnight. Then wake up to the call of breakfast waiting for you.

SERVES 2

Prep time: 5 minutes, plus overnight to let stand

Cook time: 3 minutes

½ cup chia seeds

½ teaspoon Seasonal Spice Blend (pages 60–63)

½ cup dried cherries

1 teaspoon maple syrup

1 teaspoon vanilla extract

2¼ cups Homemade Coconut Milk (page 66), divided

1. Stir the chia seeds, spice blend, and dried cherries together in a medium-size bowl.

2. In quick succession, stir in the maple syrup, vanilla, and 2 cups of coconut milk. Stir well to ensure there are no lumps.

3. Cover the bowl and let stand overnight at room temperature.

4. In the morning, heat the remaining ¼ cup of coconut milk in a saucepan over medium heat. Remove the pan from the heat. Stir in the chia pudding and warm for 1 minute before serving.

⇶ **Remedy tip** Chia seeds are astringent, a bit bitter, and good for cleansing the colon. Given that they require no cooking, they are excellent for Summer. They help calm Pitta, and can work well for Kapha, too, if made with water or Homemade Pumpkin Seed Milk (page 68) instead of coconut milk.

✿ **Season** This is a perfect Summer breakfast or snack. It is cooling and easy to prepare. If warmed, it is also a good breakfast for Winter and Spring, at which times an additional shake of ground cloves or ground ginger would be balancing.

◐ **Dosha** Pitta. For Vata, stir in ground ginger and dates when preparing, and warm with a spoonful of ghee or coconut oil before serving. For Kapha, stir in ground cloves and serve piping hot.

Breakfast Soup

ONE POT • 30 MINUTES OR LESS

At one time, breakfast for most people looked altogether different than it does now. Dinner from the night before might be reheated in the morning for what would be an ideal Ayurvedic breakfast—warm, light, nutritious. Enjoy this soup in a mug, or pour in a bowl with grains like quinoa, amaranth, or rice, as our great grandparents once did. You can also add seasonal vegetables like chopped beets, leafy greens, or roasted pumpkin, and top with toasted sesame seeds for micro crunch.

SERVES 2

Prep time: 5 minutes

Cook time: 10 minutes

2 carrots, thinly sliced

2 spring onions, thinly sliced

3 cups Basic Broth (page 59)

1 small handful dulse or another sea vegetable

1. Place the carrots, onions, broth, and dulse in a large pot and bring to a boil over high heat.

2. Reduce the heat, cover the pot, and simmer for 10 minutes. Remove from the heat.

≫ **Remedy tip** In Winter or when digestion is low, whisk a spoonful of miso in a small bowl of warm broth and pour into the soup after it is removed from the heat.

✿ **Season** Winter, Spring

❀ **Dosha** All

Breakfast Crêpes with Cinnamon-Orange Honey

With rice and beans as the primary ingredients, this delicate pancake offers a healthy dose of protein and fiber to help you start your morning strong. The orange honey syrup brightens it with a taste of sweet sunshine. It takes only a little forward planning, as you want to mix the dough the evening before to wake up to a batter ready to cook.

SERVES 4

Prep time: 5 minutes, plus 8 hours to soak and 6 hours to stand

Cook time: 25 minutes

FOR THE CRÊPES

1 cup rice

½ cup mung dal

Pinch salt (pink, mineral, or sea)

2 cups water

½ teaspoon ground cinnamon

¼ teaspoon ground cardamom

1 tablespoon Ghee (page 58), plus more as needed

FOR THE CINNAMON-ORANGE HONEY

Juice of 1 orange

¼ cup raw honey

½ teaspoon ground cinnamon

TO MAKE THE CRÊPES

1. Combine the rice and dal in a large bowl. Cover with 3 inches of water and let soak for 8 to 10 hours.

2. Drain the rice and dal, and transfer to a blender or food processor. Add the salt and water. Blend until smooth.

3. Transfer the mixture back to the bowl, cover the bowl with a towel, and let stand 6 to 12 hours, or overnight.

4. The batter should be slightly bubbly. Stir in the cinnamon and cardamom and mix well.

5. Preheat the oven to warm or its lowest setting. Melt the ghee in a large skillet over medium heat.

6. When the skillet is hot, spoon in a ladle-full of batter. Quickly swirl the batter around the pan to coat the base evenly and thinly. Cook for 2 to 3 minutes, until the crêpe is golden on the bottom. Carefully flip the crêpe and cook for 1 minute more, until both sides are golden.

7. Slide the crêpe onto a baking sheet and place it in the oven to keep warm.

8. Repeat steps 6 and 7, adding more ghee to the skillet as needed for the remaining crêpes. The batter should make 6 to 8 crêpes, depending on your skillet size.

TO MAKE THE CINNAMON-ORANGE HONEY

1. In a small bowl, whisk the orange juice with the honey and cinnamon until well blended.

2. Pour over the crêpes to serve.

⇢ **Serving tip** Pair your crêpes with half a grapefruit for a citrusy start on a Spring morning, or lather them with almond butter in Autumn. Serve the crêpes with lunch instead of bread in any season, or dip them in hummus, avocado mash, or plain yogurt for a snack. For an elegant dessert, layer each crêpe with sliced fresh fruit or spoon Seasonal Fruit Compote (page 89) over it while it cooks, drizzle with maple syrup, then fold in half and serve piping hot.

✿ **Season** Year-round

◮ **Dosha** All. For Pitta, use maple syrup instead of honey.

Buckwheat Pancakes

30 MINUTES OR LESS

These light, hearty, gluten-free pancakes are a wonderful way to introduce family and friends to Ayurveda, showing them that Ayurvedic cooking can be delicious as well as nutritious. If you don't eat eggs, replace the egg with a vegan "flax egg" (see the Ingredient tip). Cardamom is an excellent spice with buckwheat, but it can be replaced or combined with cinnamon for a more traditional taste. Coconut and almond milk are good alternatives to dairy for this batter.

SERVES 4

Prep time: 10 minutes
Cook time: 15 minutes

2 cups buckwheat flour

1 teaspoon baking powder

½ teaspoon
ground cardamom

Pinch pink salt

1 free-range egg

3½ cups milk

1 teaspoon lime zest

1 tablespoon Ghee (page 58),
plus more as needed

Maple syrup, for serving

1. Preheat the oven to its lowest setting. In a large bowl, mix the buckwheat flour with the baking powder, cardamom, and salt.

2. Whisk and stir in the egg.

3. Slowly pour in the milk, stirring constantly with a large wooden spoon until the batter has no lumps. Fold in the lime zest.

4. Melt the ghee in a small skillet. When it is hot enough that a drop of water sizzles, ladle in enough batter to cover half the bottom of the pan. Quickly swirl the batter around to coat the pan evenly and thinly. Cook for 2 minutes.

5. Flip the pancake with a spatula. Cook for about 2 minutes more, then transfer to a plate. Keep the pancakes warm in the oven until all are ready, or serve hot from the griddle.

6. Repeat steps 4 and 5 until the batter is used up. Serve with maple syrup.

>>> **Ingredient tip** To make a flax egg, stir together 1 tablespoon of ground flaxseed and 2 tablespoons of water, and let that stand for 10 minutes. Then use this as you would an egg. Flax eggs bind, but they don't rise, so they are a good substitute for eggs if you don't mind flat pancakes.

⚙ **Season** Summer, Autumn, Winter

🌢 **Dosha** Pitta. For Vata, use lemon zest instead of lime zest. For Kapha, make the batter with Homemade Pumpkin Seed Milk (page 68).

Pumpkin Nut Bread

Baking requires flour, oil, a rising agent, a binding agent, a sweetener, and seasoning. To those essentials, this recipe adds five autumnal ingredients to transform the parts into a heavenly whole. A slice of this loaf makes a delicious breakfast, especially when it's toasted and topped with yogurt and a drizzle of honey. For an open-face Summer sandwich, smear a slice with paneer, layer with cucumber slices, and top with fresh mint. In the evening, it can be a sweet dipping bread for soup or dal.

MAKES 1 LOAF

Prep time: 10 minutes

Cook time: 45 minutes

4 tablespoons ground flaxseed

½ cup water

1 cup almond flour

1 cup shredded coconut

1 tablespoon Autumn Spice Blend (page 62)

1 tablespoon psyllium husks

¼ teaspoon salt (pink, mineral, or sea)

1 teaspoon baking powder

½ cup pumpkin purée

½ cup coconut oil

¼ cup maple syrup

1 teaspoon vanilla extract

½ cup pecans

1 apple, cored and chopped

½ cup golden raisins

1. Preheat the oven to 350°F. Line an 8½-by-4½-inch loaf pan with parchment paper.

2. Make the flax eggs by mixing the flaxseed with the water in a small bowl and setting aside for 10 minutes to bind.

3. In a large bowl, mix together the almond flour, coconut, spice blend, psyllium husks, salt, and baking powder.

4. In a small bowl, whisk together the flax eggs, pumpkin, coconut oil, maple syrup, and vanilla.

5. Fold the flour mixture into the pumpkin mixture, and stir to blend thoroughly.

6. Chop the apple and mix in. Add the pecans and raisins.

7. Spoon the mixture into the loaf pan. Use a spatula to spread the batter evenly.

8. Set on the middle rack in your oven and bake for 1 hour, or until a toothpick inserted into the center of the loaf comes out clean.

>>> **Ingredient tip** Substitute molasses for maple syrup, or go half and half. For greater texture and flavor, add grated carrot or zucchini, orange zest, or chocolate chips.

❁ **Season** Summer, Autumn, Winter

◈ **Dosha** Vata, Pitta

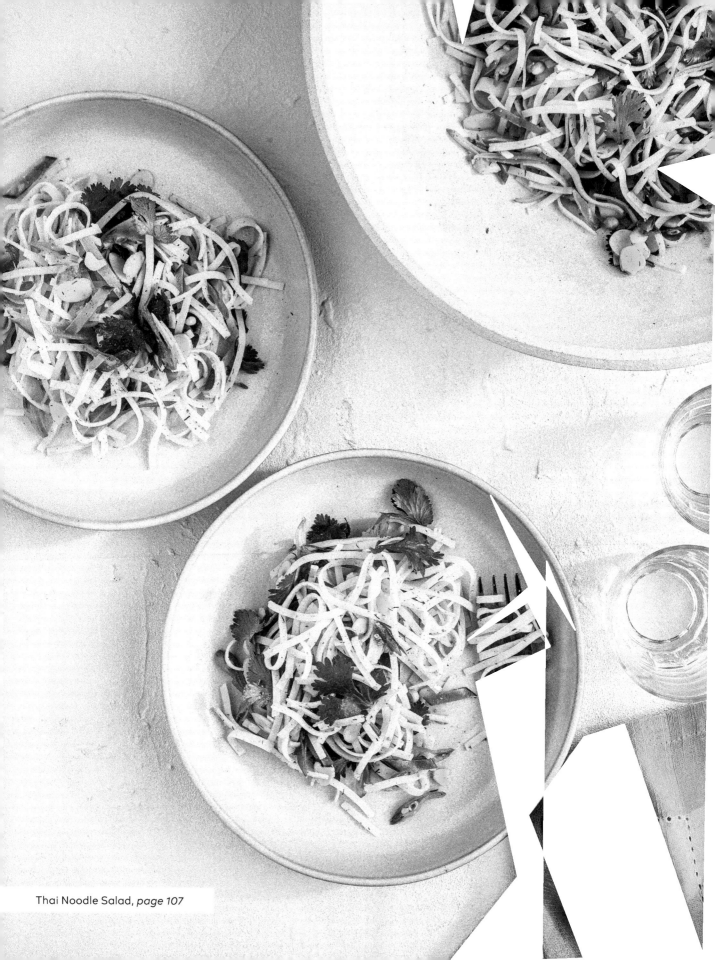

Thai Noodle Salad, *page 107*

seven
Hearty & Satisfying Lunches

Spring Kitchari 98

Asparagus & Barley Bowl 99

Spinach Paneer 100

Beans & Greens 101

Spring Pea Salad 102

Summer Kitchari 103

Berry & Peach Panzanella 104

Persian Cucumber Salad 105

Mango & Cabbage Salad 106

Thai Noodle Salad 107

Tofu Tamari Bowl 108

Roasted Vegetable Bowl 109

Autumn Kitchari 110

Sesame Noodle Stir-Fry 111

Farmer's Cheese Spread 112

Pistachio Rice with
Tahini Yogurt 113

Winter Kitchari 114

Delicious Dal 115

Winter Risotto 116

Kerala Cauliflower Stew 117

Spring Kitchari

ONE POT • KITCHEN REMEDY

Kitchari is at the core of Ayurvedic cooking, and arguably the first dish beginners learn in the Ayurvedic kitchen. The beauty of Kitchari is that it both fortifies *and* purifies. Basically a simple rice and bean dish, with the right legumes, spices, and seasonal vegetables, it becomes Ayurveda's primary healing meal. With just the right blend of macro- and micronutrients, it is deeply nourishing while easy on the digestion.

SERVES 4

Prep time: 5 minutes
Cook time: 35 minutes

½ cup basmati rice

1 cup split mung beans

1 tablespoon Ghee (page 58)

1 teaspoon mustard seeds

1 tablespoon Spring Spice Blend (page 60)

4 cups Basic Broth (page 59)

2 cups chopped vegetables, such as Spring greens, broccoli, asparagus, and snow peas

Salt (pink, mineral, or sea), for seasoning

Freshly ground black pepper

Fresh basil, for garnish

Dash red pepper flakes (optional)

1. Rinse the rice and mung beans under cool water. Set aside to drain.

2. Melt the ghee in a medium to large pot over medium heat. Stir in the mustard seeds.

3. As soon as the mustard seeds begin to pop, stir in the spice blend. Swirl the pot to blend.

4. Add the rice and mung beans, and stir to coat.

5. Add the broth. Bring to a boil, reduce the heat, cover the pot, and simmer for 20 minutes. Stir in the Spring vegetables. Cover and simmer for another 10 minutes.

6. It's done when it tastes creamy. Lightly season with salt and pepper.

7. Garnish with the basil and red pepper flakes (if using).

>>> **Remedy tip** A one-day kitchari fast helps restore your inner fires. Make one large pot, and serve with raisins for breakfast, with steamed vegetables for lunch, and with additional vegetable broth for a soupy dinner.

✿ **Season** Spring

◗ **Dosha** Kapha

Asparagus & Barley Bowl

ONE POT · KITCHEN REMEDY

In Spring when the water element is dominant (often with rain, clouds, fog, melting snow, or swollen rivers), the ingredients of this bowl—barley, asparagus, chard, and ginger—are naturally cleansing, helping us warm up and lighten up after the heaviness of Winter.

MAKES 4 SERVINGS

Prep time: 5 minutes
Cook time: 45 minutes

¾ cup barley

2 tablespoons Ghee (page 58)

1 (2-inch) piece fresh ginger, minced

2 teaspoons Spring Seasonal Blend (page 60)

6 cups Basic Broth (page 59)

1 large bunch asparagus spears, trimmed and chopped into bite-size pieces

4 leaves chard, torn into bite-size pieces

Tamari, for seasoning

1. Rinse the barley, then drain and set aside.

2. Melt the ghee in a large saucepan on medium-low heat. Add the ginger and spice blend, and sauté for 1 minute.

3. Stir in the barley. Add the broth, increase the heat, and bring to a boil. Reduce the heat to low and simmer for 40 minutes.

4. Stir in the asparagus and chard and gently simmer for 3 minutes more.

5. Taste and season with tamari.

⫸ **Serving tip** Instead of serving with crackers, try sprinkling pumpkin and sesame seeds over the soup, and consider a garnish of basil or mint for a splash of green and the fresh bite.

✿ **Season** Perfect in Spring when asparagus is fresh.

◮ **Dosha** Ideal for Kapha, who can add a hearty shake of cayenne or red pepper flakes while the soup cooks. Good for Pitta with the addition of mint and pumpkin seeds as toppings.

Spinach Paneer

30 MINUTES OR LESS

Spinach paneer has always been a favorite at my Ayurvedic cooking classes. Rich and creamy, it's like baby food for adults. If you are dairy-free, you can omit the paneer, or replace it with a soft tofu.

SERVES 2

Prep time: 15 minutes

Cook time: 10 minutes

2 cups milk

Juice of 1 lemon, divided

1 teaspoon Ghee (page 58)

1 teaspoon Seasonal Spice Blend (pages 60–63)

¼ teaspoon freshly grated nutmeg

4 cups fresh spinach, chopped

½ cup Homemade Coconut Milk (page 66)

1. In a medium pot, bring the milk to a light boil, then squeeze in half the lemon juice.

2. Remove the pot from the heat and let it sit 5 minutes while the milk solids separate.

3. Pour the milk through a cheesecloth-lined mesh strainer. Fold up the corners of the cheesecloth and twist to release all the liquid. Discard the liquid.

4. Set the cheesecloth on a plate. Put another plate on top and press down to flatten the paneer.

5. Melt the ghee in a large saucepan over medium heat. Stir in the spice blend and nutmeg, and sauté for 1 minute.

6. Add the spinach and cook for 3 minutes, stirring occasionally. Stir in the coconut milk. Reduce the heat to medium-low and simmer, uncovered, for 3 minutes.

7. Cube or crumble the paneer. Stir it into the spinach mixture. Cook for 1 minute more to warm the paneer.

8. Remove the pan from the heat. Sprinkle with the remaining lemon juice, and serve.

⇾⇾⇾ **Ingredient tip** Spinach is best when purchased in bundles rather than in boxes or bags, but be sure to clean it well. To make this dish even creamier, cook the spinach without chopping it first, and pulse the spinach mixture after step 7 in a blender. Continue with step 8.

❀ **Season** Ideal in Spring when spinach is fresh.

◑ **Dosha** Pitta, Vata. For Kapha, replace the paneer with tofu, or omit it altogether. Replace the coconut milk with vegetable broth and add red pepper flakes when sautéing the spices.

Beans & Greens

ONE POT

Beans and greens are a regular meal when I am home in my own kitchen. While the hearty warmth is especially welcome in the cooler months, staying seasonal with your greens makes this a nourishing bowl anytime of year. Expand your range with your leafy greens—rainbow chard, dandelion greens, mustard greens, watercress, and bok choy are just a few of the examples you might find at your markets—as each can add its own unique texture and flavor.

SERVES 2

Prep time: 5 minutes, plus 8 hours to soak

Cook time: 45 minutes

1 cup whole mung beans

1 teaspoon Ghee (page 58)

1 (1-inch) piece fresh ginger, peeled and minced

1 teaspoon Seasonal Spice Blend (pages 60–63)

4 cups Basic Broth (page 59)

4 cups chopped seasonal leafy greens

Salt (pink, mineral, or sea), for seasoning

Freshly ground black pepper, for seasoning

Fresh herbs, such as thyme, oregano, dill, mint, basil, cilantro, or parsley, for garnish

Roasted pumpkin seeds, for garnish

1. Put the mung beans in a bowl and cover with water. Soak for 8 hours.

2. Drain and rinse the soaked mung beans.

3. Melt the ghee in a medium saucepan over medium-high heat. Add the ginger and the spice blend and swirl the pan to mix.

4. Stir in the mung beans. Add the broth and cover the pan. Once the broth comes to a boil, cover with the lid slightly askew so a bit of steam can escape. Reduce the heat to medium-low and simmer for 20 minutes.

5. Stir in the leafy greens.

6. Reduce the heat to low and continue simmering for 10 minutes more. Taste and season with salt and black pepper. Cook until the beans are soft, then remove from the heat and let sit for 5 minutes.

7. Serve garnished with the fresh herbs and pumpkin seeds.

⫸ **Recipe tip** If you are used to a Southern pot of beans, chop sun-dried tomatoes and cook them with the beans. The tomatoes add that salty-sour, meaty taste and texture. In Autumn, serve with a spoonful of kimchi or your favorite fermented vegetables to fire up flavor and digestion.

✿ **Season** Winter, Spring, Summer

◭ **Dosha** Pitta, Kapha

Spring Pea Salad

30 MINUTES OR LESS

I love snap peas for their refreshing crunch. The snap peas contrast beautifully with the pungent and astringent tastes of radish, watercress, and cabbage in this colorful salad, whose greens, pinks, and purples celebrate the arrival of Spring.

SERVES 2

Prep time: 5 minutes

1 tablespoon mayonnaise

1 teaspoon Dijon mustard

1 teaspoon minced fresh ginger

1 tablespoon freshly squeezed lemon juice

Salt (pink, mineral, or sea), for seasoning

Freshly ground black pepper, for seasoning

2 cups fresh snap peas

1 cup shredded purple cabbage

1 radish, sliced thin

1 cup chopped watercress

1. In a small bowl, whisk together the mayonnaise, mustard, ginger, and lemon juice. Season with salt and pepper.

2. Toss the peas, cabbage, radish, and watercress together in a bowl. Drizzle with the dressing and toss to combine.

>>> **Remedy tip** For a gentle cleanse, purée the vegetables with 2 cups of vegetable broth and 1 teaspoon of ginger. Heat on the stove just to a boil. Transfer to a thermos and sip throughout the day.

❀ **Season** Spring or early Summer when snap peas are fresh.

❀ **Dosha** Pitta. For Vata and Kapha, lightly steam the vegetables before tossing them with the dressing.

Summer Kitchari

ONE POT • KITCHEN REMEDY

When Summer heat depletes us, we need a meal that is light yet substantial. We need to restore vitality, without overwhelming the digestion, and we want something simple to make, simple to serve, and simple to love. Summer Kitchari is that.

SERVES 4

Prep time: 5 minutes
Cook time: 40 minutes

1 cup basmati rice

1 cup split mung beans

1 tablespoon Ghee (page 58)

1 generous teaspoon Summer Spice Blend (page 61)

5 cups Basic Broth (page 59)

1 piece kombu or 1 hefty pinch dulse

¼ cup shredded coconut

1 cup chopped Summer vegetables, such as leafy greens, summer squash, and celery

Salt (pink, mineral, or sea), for seasoning

Freshly ground black pepper, for seasoning

Extra-virgin olive oil, for garnish

Fresh mint or cilantro, for garnish

1. Rinse the rice and mung beans under cool water. Set aside to drain.

2. Melt the ghee in a large pot over medium-high heat. Gently stir in the spice blend.

3. Add the rice and mung beans and stir to coat them with the spicy ghee.

4. Add the broth and bring to a boil.

5. Reduce the heat to low and stir in the kombu and coconut. Cover and simmer for 20 minutes.

6. Lift the lid and place the vegetables on top of the kitchari to steam. Cover and simmer for 10 minutes more.

7. Stir and taste to check that the rice and mung beans are creamy. Lightly season with salt and pepper.

8. Serve drizzled lightly with extra-virgin olive oil, and garnished with fresh mint.

≫ **Ingredient tip** Split mung beans, also called yellow dal, are the only beans that do not need to be soaked before cooking. That makes them easy to cook, while they are also famously easy on digestion. Sweet, astringent, and light, they are the perfect protein for Summer and for Pitta dosha.

❁ **Season** Summer

◬ **Dosha** Pitta

Berry & Peach Panzanella

Borrowing from the Italians, who have always understood the tasteful elegance of nature, this salad blends the juicy tart of the season's freshest stone fruits and berries with toasted bread and dandelion leaves for bright flavor. Raspberries, blackberries, or blueberries—even pomegranate—work well here. You can also use peaches, plums, apricots—play with what's available. This is a lovely brunch starter. For a special breakfast, spoon the panzanella over Breakfast Crêpes with Cinnamon-Orange Honey (page 92).

SERVES 2

Prep time: 10 minutes, plus 1 hour to marinate

2 cups torn pieces of stale or lightly toasted bread

2 cups fresh berries

2 ripe peaches, pitted and diced, juices retained

6 dandelion leaves

6 to 8 mint leaves

Juice of ½ small orange

Juice of ½ lemon

1 teaspoon champagne vinegar or white wine vinegar

1 tablespoon extra-virgin olive oil

Salt (pink, mineral, or sea), for seasoning

Freshly ground black pepper, for seasoning

Arugula, for serving

1 fresh mint sprig, for garnish

1. Put the bread, berries, and peaches with juices in a medium bowl and mix to combine.

2. Tear the dandelion and mint leaves lengthwise. Gently stir the leaves in with the bread and fruit.

3. In a small bowl, whisk together the orange juice, lemon juice, vinegar, and olive oil. Drizzle the dressing over the salad and gently toss to combine. Season with salt and pepper.

4. Cover the bowl with a plate and let stand for 1 hour for the bread to soak up the dressing and fruit juices.

5. Serve on a bed of arugula, garnished with a sprig of mint.

⇥⟩⟩ **Make-Ahead tip** Prepare in the morning and refrigerate until 1 hour before serving. Once you are ready to serve, lightly toss to see if the bread has absorbed enough of the juices. If the bread looks dry, carefully add a bit more orange juice (or lemon, vinegar, or olive oil depending on your taste), adding just enough to moisten the bread, but not too much or it will turn into a soggy mess.

✿ **Season** Late Spring/early Summer.

◭ **Dosha** Pitta. For Vata, warm the fruit and bread with 1 spoonful of ghee in a small saucepan before serving. Add a pinch of cinnamon to the dressing. For Kapha, use 1 cup of bread, and toss with ¼ teaspoon of fresh or dried oregano.

Persian Cucumber Salad

30 MINUTES OR LESS

True Ayurvedic healing meals are almost always cooked. However, after more than a decade of offering recipes, meal plans, seasonal cleanses, and resets to individual clients and groups, I have found that people of Pitta constitution really do feel refreshed and renewed after a few days of raw meals. The key is to keep it light, and make it digestible with fresh Summer herbs. This salad is one of my summer standards for Pitta, leaving them cool as a cucumber.

SERVES 2

Prep time: 10 minutes

4 medium Persian cucumbers

2 large handfuls fresh green beans

1 hefty handful arugula

½ head chopped romaine lettuce

1 cup cooked quinoa

Juice of 1 lime

2 tablespoons extra-virgin olive oil

1 bunch fresh dill

1 handful fresh cilantro

5 fresh mint leaves

Salt (pink, mineral, or sea), for seasoning

Freshly ground black pepper, for seasoning

1. Chop the cucumbers and green beans into small bite-size pieces. Toss with the arugula, romaine, and quinoa in a salad bowl.

2. Whisk the lime juice and olive oil in a small bowl. Tear the dill, cilantro, and mint and stir them into the dressing. Season with salt and pepper.

3. Drizzle the dressing over the salad and toss to combine. Serve.

⋙ **Ingredient tip** Large cucumbers, with their thick, waxy skins and bland, indigestible seeds, require peeling and often coring to be appealing, and then they lose the cleansing, toning action that comes from the astringency of seeds and skins. Persian cucumbers, with small seeds and crunchy but smooth skins, let you keep those health benefits—both the seeds and skins are deliciously digestible.

✿ **Season** Summer

△ **Dosha** Pitta

Mango & Cabbage Salad

With contrasting tastes in every bite—sweet, salty, soft, crunchy—this salad is a refreshing balance of sensations. Salting the cabbage ahead makes it tender and more digestible while intensifying its flavor and preserving its crunch. The cabbage releases its water and washes off most of the salt, so you can salt, drain, and use. But you can also rinse the cabbage and pat it dry if you are concerned about too much salt. As always, taste and proceed.

SERVES 4

Prep time: 10 minutes, plus 2 hours to drain

Cook time: 5 minutes

½ head red cabbage head, shredded

1 teaspoon salt (pink, mineral, or sea), plus more for seasoning

2 mangos

1 avocado

6 mint leaves

½ cup raw pumpkin seeds

½ teaspoon grated fresh ginger

Juice of ½ lime

1 tablespoon extra-virgin olive oil

1 teaspoon maple syrup

Freshly ground black pepper, for seasoning

1. Put the cabbage in a colander and toss it with 1 teaspoon of salt. Place the colander in the sink and allow the cabbage to drain for 2 hours.

2. Pit and cube the mangos and avocado. Tear the mint leaves into pieces.

3. Toast the pumpkin seeds in a dry pan for 1 to 5 minutes over medium heat, stirring occasionally.

4. Squeeze the liquid out of the cabbage and toss with the mangos, avocado, pumpkin seeds, and mint in a salad bowl.

5. In a small bowl, whisk together the ginger, lime juice, olive oil, and maple syrup. Taste and adjust amounts. Season with salt and pepper.

6. Drizzle the dressing over the salad and toss to combine. Serve.

⟫ **Ingredient tip** When preparing cabbage, peel off and discard the outer leaf layer. Halve lengthwise and remove the white core. For variety, mix equal amounts of red and white cabbage, or try this recipe with Napa cabbage.

❀ **Season** Ideal for Summer when the ingredients are fresh.

❀ **Dosha** Ideal for Pitta. For Vata, steam or sauté the cabbage, use lemon juice instead of lime juice in the dressing, and replace pumpkin seeds with sliced almonds. For Kapha, steam the cabbage, reduce the amount of avocado, and toss with liberal amounts of black pepper.

Thai Noodle Salad

30 MINUTES OR LESS

Cilantro is so cleansing, balancing, and cooling that it is no wonder it garnishes almost every dish in an Indian kitchen, as in many traditional cuisines around the world. Used like a leafy green, it speckles this noodle salad with emerald, signaling the fresh radiance it brings to you.

SERVES 2

Prep time: 5 minutes

Cook time: 5 minutes

1 cup snow peas

½ cup sliced almonds

1 tablespoon Ghee (page 58)

1 teaspoon Summer Spice Blend (page 61)

2 cups cooked rice noodles

1 cup cilantro

1. Slice the snow peas diagonally into thin strips.

2. Toast the almonds in a dry pan over medium heat for 2 minutes.

3. Add the ghee, and once it is melted, stir in the spice blend and sauté for 1 minute.

4. Toss the noodles and peas with the ghee, spices, and almond slices.

5. Remove the pan from the heat and lightly stir in the cilantro.

Remedy tip Cilantro is a powerful purifier and Pitta pacifier. It is strongly astringent and bitter, so when cooking with it, consider the sweet taste of rice or coconut to provide balance. For liver support, make a tonic by blending handfuls of it, stems and all, with coconut water or plain water. Strain and drink. The pulp can be used topically as a poultice to help calm irritable skin rashes.

Season Summer, Autumn

Dosha Pitta. For Vata, use the Autumn Spice Blend (page 62).

Tofu Tamari Bowl

ONE POT • 30 MINUTES OR LESS

Most ancient cultures evolved digestible and deliciously healthy dietary models. Ayurveda emerged from India and is therefore associated with the Indian kitchen, but we also can find Ayurvedic principles in many dishes throughout the world. Japan, for instance, has a culinary tradition almost perfectly adapted for Pitta dosha. That tradition is embodied in this refreshingly simple, elegant, and nourishing bowl.

SERVES 2

Prep time: 5 minutes

Cook time: 5 minutes

1 teaspoon Ghee (page 58)

1 teaspoon Summer Spice Blend (page 61)

1 cup snap peas

2 cups cubed soft tofu

1 tablespoon sesame seeds

1 cup Basic Broth (page 59)

1 tablespoon tamari

1. Melt the ghee in a medium saucepan over medium-high heat. Stir in the spice blend.

2. Add the peas and sauté for 1 minute.

3. Add the tofu, sesame seeds, and broth, and gently simmer, uncovered, for 1 minute more.

4. Remove the pan from the heat and stir in the tamari. Serve.

⋙ **Serving tip** Garnish with cilantro and pumpkin seeds for the added health benefits, color, and crunch.

✿ **Season** Summer

◓ **Dosha** Pitta. For Kapha, use the Spring Spice Blend (page 60), add red pepper flakes to the spices, and reduce the amount of tamari to 1 teaspoon. For Vata, use the Autumn Spice Blend (page 62) and toss with cooked rice.

Roasted Vegetable Bowl

30 MINUTES OR LESS

If you have a spiralizer, you can have fun making noodles out of root vegetables. Once roasted, the noodles go surprisingly well with fresh lettuce for a hearty play of sweet and crisp in a late-Summer salad. If you don't have a spiralizer, you can use a mandoline to make thin slices that will roast up quickly and caramelly, or chop into matchsticks. Choose from the root vegetables you find at your market. Sweet potatoes, yams, beets, parsnips, turnips—all are delicious roasted and make a colorful bowl when served together.

SERVES 2

Prep time: 5 minutes
Cook time: 20 minutes

3 root vegetables

1 tablespoon Ghee (page 58)

1 teaspoon Seasonal Spice Blend (pages 60–63)

Salt (pink, mineral, or sea), for seasoning

Freshly ground black pepper, for seasoning

1 tablespoon freshly squeezed lemon juice

1. Preheat the oven to 475°F. Line a baking sheet with parchment paper.

2. Lightly scrub the vegetables. If you have a spiralizer, make noodles out of the root vegetables. (Otherwise, slice them into matchstick-size pieces.) Put the vegetables in a large bowl.

3. Melt the ghee over medium heat. Stir in the spice blend. Pour the spiced ghee over the vegetables. Toss to combine.

4. Spread the vegetables in a single layer across the baking sheet. Roast until the vegetables begin to brown, about 10 minutes.

5. Turn the vegetables and roast for another 3 minutes, until a sweet aroma rises from the oven.

6. Remove the vegetables from the oven, and sprinkle with salt and pepper. Allow to cool slightly.

7. Splash with the lemon juice and serve immediately.

>>> **Serving tip** In Summer, serve over a bed of gem lettuce or arugula, or toss with microgreens. In Autumn, serve with Tahini Yogurt (page 113), or simply a spoonful of ghee and fresh herbs.

Season Ideal for late Summer. In Autumn and Winter, serve with sautéed greens.

Dosha Vata, Pitta. For Kapha, serve with steamed greens and red pepper flakes.

Autumn Kitchari

ONE POT • KITCHEN REMEDY

Autumn's shorter days, colder nights, and drying winds can leave us feeling depleted. This is the ideal time for kitchari—a warm, sweet, lightly spiced, easily digested, and nutritious food—ideal for a season when comfort is prescribed.

SERVES 4

Prep time: 5 minutes

Cook time: 40 minutes

1 cup basmati rice

½ cup split mung beans

2 tablespoons Ghee (page 58)

1 generous teaspoon Autumn Spice Blend (page 62)

5 cups Basic Broth (page 59)

1 cup Homemade Coconut Milk (page 66)

1 (1-inch) piece kombu

1 cup chopped Autumn vegetables, such as carrots, beets, and celery

Tamari, for seasoning

Fresh mint or basil, for garnish

1. Rinse the rice and mung beans under cool water. Set aside to drain.

2. Melt the ghee in a large pot over medium heat. Stir in the spice blend.

3. Add the rice and beans. Stir to coat with the spiced ghee.

4. Add the broth and coconut milk, and bring to a boil.

5. Reduce the heat to low. Stir in the kombu. Cover the pot and simmer for 20 minutes.

6. Lift the lid and stir in the vegetables. Cover and simmer for 15 minutes more.

7. Stir and taste to check if the rice and beans are creamy.

8. Serve with a drizzle of tamari and a garnish of fresh mint or basil.

>>> **Serving tip** Change it up by making it goopy with ghee, raita, fermented vegetables, or an extra cup of hot broth.

✿ **Season** Autumn

🍃 **Dosha** Vata

Sesame Noodle Stir-Fry

30 MINUTES OR LESS

This stir-fry is tossed with a creamy almond butter sauce that makes the sauté sing, and turns this noodle dish into one of my autumn cravings.

SERVES 2

Prep time: 5 minutes

Cook time: 10 minutes

1 (8-ounce) package soba noodles

2 tablespoons Ghee (page 58)

1 teaspoon Autumn Spice Blend (page 62)

2 carrots, shredded

1 teaspoon minced fresh ginger

1 head bok choy, trimmed and thinly sliced crosswise

½ cup sesame seeds

1 tablespoon almond butter

1 teaspoon shoyu or tamari

⅛ teaspoon garlic powder

1 tablespoon hot water

Salt (pink, mineral, or sea), for seasoning

Freshly ground black pepper, for seasoning

Extra-virgin olive oil, for drizzling

1. In a large bowl, pour hot water over the soba noodles and set aside.

2. Melt the ghee in a skillet over medium-high heat. Stir in the spice blend and swirl the pan to combine.

3. Add the carrots and ginger and cook for 2 minutes, stirring frequently.

4. Stir in the bok choy and sesame seeds. Reduce the heat to medium and cook for 3 minutes.

5. In a small bowl, whisk together the almond butter, shoyu, and garlic powder with the hot water.

6. Drain the noodles. Add them to the pan with the vegetables. Pour in the dressing and toss to combine.

7. Season with the salt and pepper, and serve with a drizzle of olive oil.

Serving tip Garnish with cilantro or fresh mint.

Seasons Autumn

Dosha Vata. For Pitta, omit the garlic powder and replace the almond butter with pumpkin seed butter.

Farmer's Cheese Spread

Farmer's cheese is made by separating yogurt into curds and whey. The curds can be whisked into a cottage cheese or pressed into a paneer. In this case, they are blended into a creamy soft spread. Full of probiotics, it's a sweet-sour taste combination that is excellent for Vata, and for Autumn meals. You can spread it on crackers, or toast for a sandwich, or press it into a block to make paneer, which then can be crumbled and stirred in with saag, sautéed greens, curry, or any sauté.

MAKES ABOUT 2 CUPS

Prep time: 5 minutes, plus 2 hours to drain

1 (1-quart) container full-fat yogurt

1 pinch salt (pink, mineral, or sea)

1 teaspoon extra-virgin olive oil

1. Line a strainer with a large piece of cheesecloth or a thin kitchen towel and set the strainer inside a large bowl. Pour the yogurt into the strainer and let it sit for 1 hour at room temperature.

2. Lift the edges of the cheesecloth, draw the corners together, and twist. Tie a knot close to the yogurt. Remove the strainer and hang the cheesecloth above the bowl. Let it drain for 1 hour more.

3. What remains in the cheesecloth is the farmer's cheese. Put it in a large bowl and sprinkle it with salt and olive oil.

4. Refrigerate in an airtight container for up to 5 days.

>>> **Ingredient tip** The liquid that remains in the bowl is whey. The whey can be saved in a glass jar in the refrigerator to make fermented vegetables, or stirred right into a bowl of soup, or mixed with an equal part of warm water and sipped for a probiotic tonic.

✿ **Seasons** Autumn

♨ **Dosha** Vata

Pistachio Rice with Tahini Yogurt

30 MINUTES OR LESS

This is a great lunch to pack for days when you are on the go. You can spoon the yogurt into the bottom of a mason jar, layer the rice above, and garnish with parsley and mint on top, then turn upside down and pour into a bowl at lunchtime. It's also a great complement to the Delicious Dal (page 115), and is light and refreshing on a bed of buttery greens.

SERVES 2

Prep time: 5 minutes

Juice of 2 lemons, divided

¼ cup extra-virgin olive oil

1 cup cooked basmati rice

¼ cup pistachios

½ cup fresh mint

Salt (pink, mineral, or sea), for seasoning

Freshly ground black pepper, for seasoning

½ cup whole-milk yogurt

¼ cup water

¼ cup tahini

½ teaspoon ground ginger

½ teaspoon ground cumin

1 cup chopped fresh parsley

1. In a medium bowl, whisk the juice of 1 lemon with the olive oil.

2. Stir in the rice, pistachios, and mint. Season with salt and pepper.

3. In a small bowl, whisk the yogurt, water, tahini, the remaining lemon juice, the ginger, and the cumin. Stir in the parsley. Season with salt and pepper.

4. Spoon the tahini yogurt over the rice and serve.

⇉ **Ingredient tip** This works especially well with a less starchy rice like red rice, black rice, or wild rice.

✿ **Season** Autumn

◬ **Dosha** Vata

Winter Kitchari

KITCHEN REMEDY

Kitchari is an Ayurvedic staple—balancing, tonifying, and cleansing—and so welcoming in Winter as a bowl of piping-hot, full-spectrum nutrition. This is full-body delicious: Home-cooked kitchari awakens cellular intelligence to the point where you can almost hear your body hum.

SERVES 4

Prep time: 5 minutes
Cook time: 40 minutes

1 cup basmati rice

1 cup split mung beans

1 tablespoon Ghee (page 58)

1 generous teaspoon Winter Spice Blend (page 63)

4 cups Basic Broth (page 59)

2 cups water

1 cup chopped Winter vegetables, such as carrots, celery, broccoli, cauliflower, or kale

2 tablespoons sesame seeds

Salt (pink, mineral, or sea), for seasoning

Freshly ground black pepper, for seasoning

Shoyu or tamari, for drizzling

Fresh rosemary, thyme, or basil for garnish

1. Rinse the rice and mung beans under cool water. Set aside to drain.

2. Melt the ghee in a large pot over medium heat. Gently stir in the spice blend.

3. Add the rice and mung beans, and stir to coat with the spicy ghee.

4. Add the broth and water, and bring to a boil. Reduce the heat, stir the rice and beans, cover the pot, and simmer for 20 minutes.

5. Lift the lid and place the vegetables on top of the rice and mung beans to steam. Cover the pot again and simmer 10 minutes more.

6. Toast the sesame seeds in a small pan for 3 minutes over medium heat, stirring frequently. Taste to see if the rice and beans are tender. Lightly season with salt and pepper.

7. Sprinkle on the sesame seeds and drizzle the shoyu. Serve garnished with the fresh herbs.

>>> **Remedy tip** Think of kitchari as Ayurveda's version of chicken soup, and therefore perfect for Winter's seasonal chills. Make it weekly to be proactive. Serve it daily when recuperating.

✿ **Season** Winter

❧ **Dosha** Vata, Kapha

Delicious Dal

ONE POT · 30 MINUTES OR LESS

This savory dal is made from split mung beans, also called yellow dal. When split, mung beans are light, easy to digest, high in protein, and high in fiber—an Ayurvedic healing staple, and they cook up quickly without any need for presoaking.

MAKES 2 SERVINGS

Prep time: 5 minutes
Cook time: 25 minutes

1 cup split mung beans

1 tablespoon Ghee (page 58)

½ teaspoon brown or yellow mustard seeds

1 teaspoon Seasonal Spice Blend (pages 60–63)

3 cups Basic Broth (page 59)

Salt (pink, mineral, or sea), for seasoning

Freshly ground black pepper, for seasoning

1. Rinse and drain the mung beans.

2. Melt the ghee in a medium pot over medium heat. Add the mustard seeds and sauté until they begin to pop.

3. Add the spice blend and swirl to mix.

4. Stir in the mung beans.

5. Add the broth and bring it to a gentle boil.

6. Reduce the heat to low, cover the pot, and simmer for 20 minutes, or until the beans are cooked through.

7. Season with salt and pepper.

⇒⟩⟩ **Serving tip** While this is delicious on its own, you can make it heartier with rice or quinoa, and with a vegetable such as chopped chard or steamed squash. A spoonful of ghee or coconut oil stirred into your serving, and shoyu or tamari instead of salt, really enriches. Garnish with cilantro.

⇒⟩⟩ **Ingredient tip** Split mung beans can be difficult to find; call your local Indian/Asian market, or order online from one of the sellers listed in the Resources (page 204). Otherwise, whole mung beans will work; they just need to be soaked for 8 to 10 hours, and take twice the time to cook.

✿ **Season** Year-round

◓ **Dosha** All

Winter Risotto

ONE POT • 30 MINUTES OR LESS

Usually prepared with a short-grain Arborio rice, risotto can be made healthier by using the lower glycemic and lesser calorie basmati rice. For a cheesy version, stir in 1 tablespoon of Parmesan cheese when the rice is cooked and before seasoning with salt and pepper. Or, as suggested in the tip, serve with paneer. For a cheesy vegan version, stir in 1–2 tablespoons nutritional yeast.

SERVES 4

Prep time: 5 minutes

Cook time: 20 minutes

2 tablespoons Ghee (page 58)

1 celery stalk, minced

1 cup basmati rice

1 tablespoon lemon zest

Juice of 1 lemon

5 cups Basic Broth (page 59), divided

1 cup finely chopped seasonal greens

Salt (pink, mineral, or sea), for seasoning

Freshly ground black pepper, for seasoning

1. Heat the ghee in a large saucepan over medium heat. Add the celery and cook for 2 minutes. Add the rice and sauté, stirring constantly, for 2 minutes. Add the lemon zest and juice, and cook, stirring gently and vigilantly, till the liquid has been absorbed.

2. Add 1 cup of broth to the pan and stir until the broth is absorbed. Continue adding another 1 cup of broth in ½-cup amounts, always stirring until it is absorbed. When you've stirred in 2 cups of broth, add the greens, then continue adding the broth in ½-cup increments.

3. When all the broth is added and absorbed and the rice is tender, season it with salt and pepper, and serve.

Serving tip Serve with cubes of Paneer (page 100) and fresh thyme, oregano, or basil, a drizzle of extra-virgin olive oil, and generous turns of the pepper mill.

Season Winter

Dosha Vata, Pitta

Kerala Cauliflower Stew

ONE POT · 30 MINUTES OR LESS

This is a colorful pot of Winter bounty. Great for casual meals with friends and family, it is a celebration of the winter hearth. In addition to the vegetables listed, include the best of market-fresh vegetables—broccolini, snap peas, celery, leafy greens, zucchini, turnips, or whatever is in season. This stew always nourishes and satisfies.

SERVES 4

Prep time: 5 minutes
Cook time: 20 minutes

1 tablespoon Ghee (page 58)

2 tablespoons Winter Spice Blend (page 63)

1 head cauliflower, cut into bite-size florets

2 cups chopped green beans

2 carrots, chopped into bite-size pieces

6 cups Basic Broth (page 59)

1½ cups Homemade Coconut Milk (page 66)

Salt (pink, mineral, or sea), for seasoning

Freshly ground black pepper, for seasoning

1. Melt the ghee in a large pot over medium-low heat. Add the spice blend and sauté for 1 minute.

2. Stir in the cauliflower, green beans, and carrots, and sauté for 3 minutes.

3. Add the broth and bring to a boil. Cover the pot and reduce the heat to low. Simmer for 10 minutes.

4. Stir in the coconut milk. Simmer for 3 minutes more so the flavors integrate.

5. Season with salt and pepper.

⇉ **Serving tip** Garnish each serving with toasted nuts or seeds, and fresh herbs like basil or oregano.

❀ **Season** Winter. Modify for any season with seasonal spices and vegetables.

◬ **Dosha** All, with appropriate seasonal spice blends.

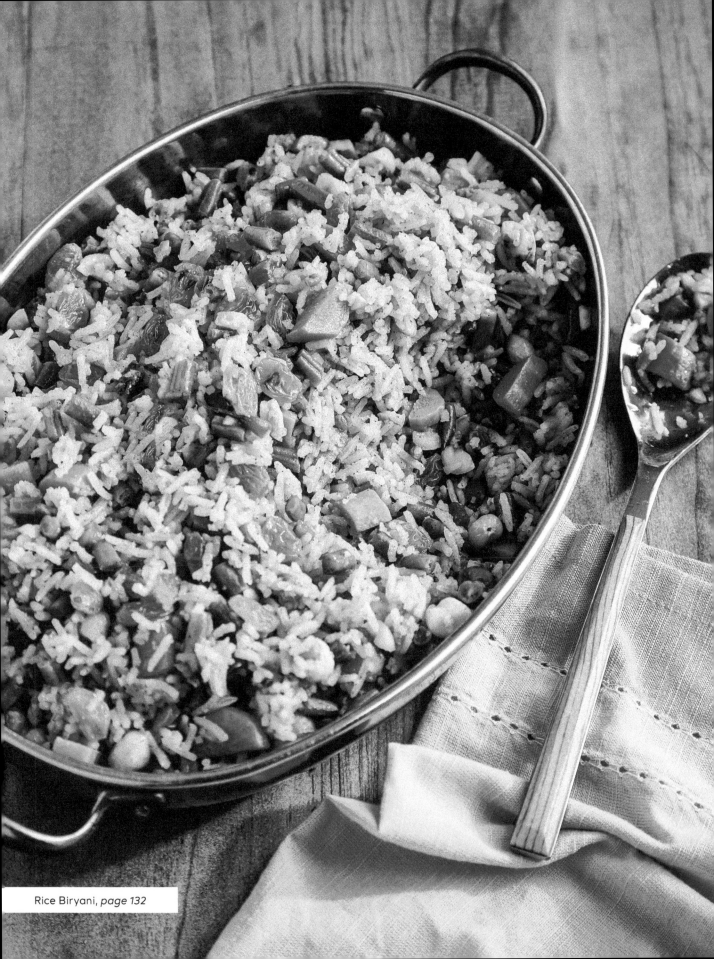

Rice Biryani, *page 132*

eight
Light & Simple Dinners

Mung Bean Soup 120

Restorative Roots
& Shoots Broth 121

Miso Soup with Asparagus 122

Creamy Watercress Soup 123

Simple Saag 124

Ginger Broccolini 125

Mint Pea Soup 126

Summer Gazpacho 127

Coconut Squash Dal 128

Roasted Roots Ecrasse 129

Asian Noodle Soup 130

Ginger-Carrot Soup 131

Rice Biryani 132

Pho Soup 134

Curried Green Beans 135

Borscht 136

Fennel & Fava Bean Soup 138

Seasonal Vegetable Purée 140

Healing Kanji 141

Mung Bean Soup

ONE POT · KITCHEN REMEDY

Mung beans are Ayurvedic beauties—sweet, light, and astringent. Cooked with ghee and broth to balance the dryness of the astringency, and with pungent spices to improve digestibility, this soup can be garnished with cilantro for a six-taste wholeness. It is delicious any day of the week, and particularly healing when healing is needed.

SERVES 2

Prep time: 5 minutes, plus 8 hours to soak

Cook time: 45 minutes

1 cup whole mung beans

1 tablespoon Ghee (page 58)

1 (1-inch) piece fresh ginger, peeled and minced

1 teaspoon Seasonal Spice Blend (pages 60–63)

6 cups Basic Broth (page 59)

1 cup leafy greens, finely chopped

1. Put the mung beans in a bowl and cover with water. Soak for 8 hours.

2. Rinse and drain the mung beans.

3. Melt the ghee in a large pot over medium-high heat. Add the ginger and the spice blend, and swirl the pot to coat.

4. Stir in the mung beans. Add the broth and cover the pot. Bring to a low boil, then reduce the heat to medium. Cook for 30 minutes.

5. Stir in the greens. Cook another 10 minutes, or until the beans are soft.

>>> **Serving tip** Toast a handful of coconut flakes and pumpkin seeds for 3 minutes in a dry pan and use as a topping along with fresh cilantro.

✿ **Season** Year-round

❀ **Dosha** All

Restorative Roots & Shoots Broth

ONE POT • 30 MINUTES OR LESS • KITCHEN REMEDY

In the Japanese tradition of macrobiotics, there is a healing broth made from a "round, a root, and a shoot." The round could be an onion, a beet, garlic, or an apple. The root could be a carrot, sweet potato, daikon radish, or ginger; the shoot is something that grows above ground like celery, kale, chard, spinach, or bok choy. The idea is that you get the energies of above and below, and all around to aid you in your healing. Keep this broth in a thermos and sip all day as a restorative tea, or enjoy it as a soup for dinner whenever your digestive fire is low.

SERVES 2

Prep time: 5 minutes

Cook time: 20 minutes

1 beet

1 daikon radish

1 celery stalk

4 cups water

Pinch salt
(pink, mineral, or sea)

Pinch freshly ground
black pepper

1. Roughly chop the beet, radish, and celery.

2. Place the vegetables in a soup pot with the water and the salt and pepper.

3. Bring to a boil, then reduce the heat to low and simmer for 15 minutes.

4. Strain and serve.

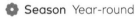 **Remedy tip** Sweet, pungent, astringent, and bitter in taste, this is a deeply restorative healing broth. Add a 1-inch piece of peeled fresh ginger to the cooking, and season with apple cider vinegar or tamari to boost the benefits to digestion and immunity.

 Season Year-round

Dosha Vata

Miso Soup with Asparagus

30 MINUTES OR LESS • KITCHEN REMEDY

Miso soup comes from the Japanese tradition, where it is heralded for its healing power. It is not typically Ayurvedic, yet it embodies the Ayurvedic principles for an evening meal—light, warm, easily digested, *sattvic*. The broth alone is so Vata pacifying that it could double as a soothing tea in the afternoon hours when Vata rises. This recipe adds soft tofu and crunchy asparagus to balance all six tastes for a comforting soup that satisfies.

SERVES 4

Prep time: 5 minutes

Cook time: 20 minutes

5 cups Basic Broth (page 59)

2 teaspoons grated fresh ginger

1 bunch asparagus, trimmed and chopped

1 cup cubed soft tofu

3 tablespoons light-colored miso

Tamari, for seasoning

1. Bring the broth to a boil in a large saucepan over medium-high heat. Stir in the ginger.

2. Reduce the heat to low. Cover the pan and simmer for 10 minutes.

3. Add the asparagus and tofu to the broth and return the liquid to a simmer. Cook for 3 to 5 minutes, until the asparagus is just tender.

4. Turn off the heat. Ladle ¼ cup of the broth into a bowl and add the miso. Whisk to combine, then stir back into the soup.

5. Taste and season with tamari. Serve hot.

Remedy tip Skip the asparagus and tofu to make a warm Vata-reducing broth that can be sipped like tea throughout the day, or stirred with rice for a sweet, easy meal.

Season Perfect for Spring, when asparagus is fresh. It is also good in Winter when you can replace the asparagus with green beans.

Dosha For Kapha, serve with a sprinkle of red pepper flakes. For Vata, replace the asparagus with shredded carrots. For Pitta, use half the amount of miso.

Creamy Watercress Soup

30 MINUTES OR LESS

Purifying and light, this elegant emerald soup is perfect for Spring, when fresh watercress is abundant. With pungent, astringent, and bitter as its dominant tastes, watercress soup is ideal in this season of Kapha. If available, a leaf of lemongrass added to the pot while cooking evokes a sweet hint of South Asia. Otherwise, thyme, basil, dill, or a generous drizzle of Hot & Spicy Oil (page 64) adds a good flavor edge.

MAKES 2 SERVINGS

Prep time: 5 minutes

Cook time: 10 minutes

1 teaspoon Ghee (page 58)

1 teaspoon minced fresh ginger

1 teaspoon Spring Spice Blend (page 60)

2 cups watercress

2 cups spinach

2 cups water

1 cup Homemade Coconut Milk (page 66)

Salt (pink, mineral, or sea), for seasoning

Freshly ground black pepper, for seasoning

1. Melt the ghee in a soup pot over medium heat. Stir in the ginger and the spice blend, and sauté for 1 minute.

2. Add the watercress, spinach, and water, and bring to a gentle boil. Cook for 3 minutes.

3. Pour the mixture into a blender, or use an immersion blender, and pulse to purée the soup.

4. Return the soup to the pot over medium-low heat and stir in the coconut milk. Cook for 3 minutes.

5. Season with salt and pepper, and serve.

>>> **Serving tip** Serve with a drizzle of extra-virgin olive oil. Garnish with parsley for Kapha; cilantro, or mint for Pitta; and coconut flakes or chopped pine nuts for Vata.

Season Spring

Dosha Kapha. For Pitta, use Summer Spice Blend (page 61). For Vata, reduce the amount of watercress to 1 cup, or omit it altogether and just make spinach soup; use the Autumn Spice Blend (page 62).

Simple Saag

30 MINUTES OR LESS

Saag is traditionally made with mustard greens, spinach, and fenugreek leaves to create a Spring balance of bitter, astringent, pungent, and semi-sweet tastes. Fenugreek leaves, also called *methi*, are ideal, but can be substituted with watercress or celery leaves. In fact, all the greens can be substituted with whatever greens are seasonally available to you. I often add beet greens, kale, chard, dandelion leaves, or even a bit of arugula. Just be sure to balance bitter greens evenly with a milder green, like spinach. Fresh paneer is crumbled in to balance the light and rough of the greens with sweet and creamy.

SERVES 2

Prep time: 5 minutes

Cook time: 10 minutes

2 tablespoons Ghee (page 58)

2 teaspoons Spring Spice Blend (page 60)

1 teaspoon fresh, minced ginger

2 cups chopped fresh spinach

2 cups chopped mustard greens

1 cup chopped fresh fenugreek leaves

¼ cup Basic Broth (page 59) or water

¼ cup crumbled fresh Paneer (page 100)

Freshly squeezed lemon juice, for drizzling

Salt (pink, mineral, or sea), for seasoning

Freshly ground black pepper, for seasoning

1. In a large skillet, heat the ghee over medium heat. Stir in the spice blend and ginger and sauté for 1 minute.

2. Add the spinach, mustard greens, and fenugreek leaves, and stir thoroughly, coating the greens in the spicy ghee. Reduce the heat to low, cover the skillet, and cook until the greens are thoroughly wilted, stirring occasionally, about 5 minutes.

3. Transfer the mixture to a blender with the broth. Pulse 3 times. (You want only to get a fine chop, not turn it into soup.)

4. Transfer back to the skillet. Stir the paneer into the saag.

5. Drizzle with the lemon juice, and season with salt and pepper.

>>> **Serving tip** Paneer can be replaced with silken tofu. Saag can be served with rice, over toast, tossed with pasta, or nestled in the veggies from Roasted Vegetable Bowl (page 109).

Season Spring. Appropriate for Summer with spinach and Summer leafy greens instead of Spring greens.

Dosha Kapha. For Pitta, use Summer Spice Blend (page 61), replace the fresh ginger with 1 teaspoon of ground ginger, reduce the amount of mustard greens, and optionally replace the broth with Homemade Coconut Milk (page 66). For Vata, cook in 1 cup of milk plus a hearty pinch nutmeg, and serve over rice.

Ginger Broccolini

30 MINUTES OR LESS • KITCHEN REMEDY

There is a saying that "cancer hates cabbage." In fact, cancer hates the entire cabbage family, the Brassicas, whose kin include broccoli, cauliflower, collards, kale, bok choy, Brussels sprouts, mustard greens, and watercress. Prepared with pungent spices, this Ginger Broccolini is light, astringent, and bitter, making it also deliciously brilliant for balancing Kapha.

SERVES 2

Prep time: 5 minutes

Cook time: 10 minutes

1 bunch broccolini

1 tablespoon Ghee (page 58)

1 tablespoon minced fresh ginger

1 teaspoon lemon zest

1 tablespoon freshly squeezed lemon juice

Salt (pink, mineral, or sea), for seasoning

Freshly ground black pepper, for seasoning

1. Bring a large pot of salted water to a boil. Fill a large bowl with water and ice.

2. Add the broccolini to the pot and cook for 2 minutes.

3. Drain the broccolini and immediately immerse it in the bowl of ice water.

4. Melt the ghee in a large skillet over medium heat. Stir in the ginger and zest.

5. Drain the broccolini and add it to the skillet. Cook for 2 minutes.

6. Remove the pan from the heat. Drizzle in the lemon juice and toss to combine. Season with salt and pepper, and serve.

Ingredient tip In Summer, cook the broccolini with a sliced fennel bulb for a sweet-bitter combination of tastes.

Season Ideal in Spring. Also good in Winter, Summer.

Dosha Kapha. For Pitta, replace the lemon juice with lime juice, and (optionally) the ginger with ½ teaspoon of fennel seeds.

Mint Pea Soup

Fresh peas in Spring are nothing like the frozen and boiled peas so many people are used to. This soup is creamy and rich, and the flavor comes alive with fresh mint. In Spring, it is purifying and light for dinner. In Summer, it is cool with coconut milk and best served at room temperature.

SERVES 6

Prep time: 5 minutes
Cook time: 10 minutes

2 tablespoons Ghee (page 58)

1 teaspoon Spring Spice Blend (page 60)

4 cups Basic Broth (page 59)

5 cups freshly shelled peas

½ cup chopped fresh mint leaves

1 cup pumpkin seeds

Salt (pink, mineral, or sea), for seasoning

Freshly ground black pepper, for seasoning

½ cup chopped fresh parsley

1. Heat the ghee in a large saucepan over medium-low heat, add the spice blend, and cook for 1 minute.

2. Add the broth. Increase the heat to high and bring to a boil.

3. Add the peas and cook for 4 minutes, or until the peas are tender.

4. Remove the pan from the heat. Stir in the mint leaves and pumpkin seeds.

5. Transfer the soup to a blender, or use an immersion blender, and purée the soup. Season with salt and pepper.

6. Serve hot with a generous topping of parsley.

Ingredient tip To shuck fresh peas, hold the pod in your hand. Turn it on its side, and press your thumb on its seam, squeezing lengthwise to pop open the pod. Run a finger down the inside of the pod to free the peas and let them run into a waiting bowl.

Season Spring. For Summer, use the Summer Spice Blend (page 61), add 1 cup of coconut milk to the purée, and serve at room temperature.

Dosha Kapha. Pitta, with Summer adjustments.

Summer Gazpacho

30 MINUTES OR LESS

This is not technically a gazpacho, which despite being refreshing on a Summer day is full of nightshades and therefore not advised for Pitta or in the Summer season. Still, this room-temperature soup achieves the chunky freshness of gazpacho with a blend of Summer's most cooling ingredients. Eat slowly so you can taste all the flavors. They are complex and delicious!

SERVES 2

Prep time: 5 minutes

1 cucumber, cut into about 4 pieces

1 zucchini, cut into about 4 pieces

1 handful cherry tomatoes

1 small avocado, pitted

1 handful Summer herbs, such as dill, cilantro, fennel fronds, or basil

Freshly squeezed lime juice, for drizzling

Mint leaves, for garnish

1. Put the cucumber, zucchini, cherry tomatoes, avocado, and herbs in a blender and pulse just a few times, until you get a chunky consistency.

2. Serve in bowls. Drizzle with lime juice and garnish with mint.

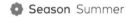 **Preparation tip** Do not add ice, as some Summer soups do. No matter how hot the temperature, ice only slows digestion. In Summer, room temperature is best—for drinks as well as soups.

Season Summer

Dosha Pitta

Coconut Squash Dal

ONE POT • 30 MINUTES OR LESS • KITCHEN REMEDY

Dal is a hulled, split legume, of which there are many varieties, including mung dal, which is green when whole but light yellow when hulled and split. *Dal* is also a term that refers to the dish made from legumes, and this recipe gives you mung bean manna, with melt-in-your-mouth squash and milky coconut. Choose from kale, collards, or chard for hearty greens that hold up while helping keep Pitta down.

SERVES 2

Prep time: 5 minutes

Cook time: 25 minutes

1 cup split mung beans

1 tablespoon Ghee (page 58)

1 teaspoon Summer Spice Blend (page 61)

1 cup cubed seasonal squash

2 cups chopped leafy greens

3 cups Basic Broth (page 59)

1 cup Homemade Coconut Milk (page 66)

Tamari, for seasoning

1. Rinse the mung beans under cool water and set aside to drain.

2. Melt the ghee in a large pot over medium heat. Stir in the spice blend and sauté for 1 minute.

3. Add the mung beans, squash, and greens, and stir until they're thoroughly coated in the spicy ghee. Sauté for 1 minute.

4. Increase the heat to high and add the broth. Bring to a boil, then cover the pot and reduce the heat to low. Simmer for 20 minutes.

5. Stir in the coconut milk and bring the pot back to a simmer. Cook for 1 minute more.

6. Season with tamari and serve.

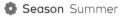 **Serving tip** For a garnish with a light crunch, toast a handful of shredded coconut, coconut flakes, or pumpkin seeds. Or garnish with cilantro, parsley, basil, or all three.

✿ **Season** Summer

🔺 **Dosha** Pitta

Roasted Roots Ecrasse

KITCHEN REMEDY

Ecrasse is a fancy word for mash. Think of this as a healthier version of mashed potatoes. Carrots, sweet potatoes, beets, turnips, and rutabagas are all delicious roasted and mashed, but my favorite is parsnips. Parsnip makes a creamy cloud of nourishment with just a light, pungent edge. Like any good mash, this is delicious seasoned simply with salt and freshly ground black pepper, or served with a hot pour of the vegetarian gravy from the Gravy & Mash recipe (page 153).

SERVES 2

Prep time: 10 minutes

Cook time: 45 minutes

2 of a root vegetable, such as carrots, sweet potatoes, beets, turnips, rutabagas, or parsnips

1 tablespoon Ghee (page 58)

½ cup Homemade Coconut Milk (page 66), plus more as needed

1 teaspoon Autumn Spice Blend (page 62)

Salt (pink, mineral, or sea), for seasoning

Freshly ground black pepper, for seasoning

1. Preheat the oven to 475°F.

2. Prick each vegetable two or three times with a fork. Place the vegetables on a baking sheet.

3. Roast for 45 minutes, or until a knife slides through easily. Remove from the oven and let cool for 5 minutes.

4. Peel the vegetables and put them in a blender with the ghee, coconut milk, and spice blend. Blend to a creamy consistency.

5. Season with salt and pepper.

>>> **Ingredient tip** To prick or not to prick? Some people like to prick holes in a root vegetable before roasting it, to release steam and prevent a soggy tuber. Others say that no prick creates a creamier outcome. My invitation is to experiment and see what works best for you.

⚙ **Season** Autumn

◬ **Dosha** Vata, Pitta

Asian Noodle Soup

30 MINUTES OR LESS

Soups are warm, hydrating, and restorative on Autumn nights as the winds rise and darkness descends. This simple noodle soup is easy to make, and easy to love for its slurpy savory warmth. Rice noodles are sweet, spinach is bitter, ginger is pungent, and tamari is salty/sour, giving you all but the driest of tastes, astringent, for a comforting Vata-balancing meal. Stir in soft tofu for added protein—and the astringent taste that completes the six-taste wholeness.

SERVES 2

Prep time: 5 minutes

Cook time: 20 minutes

1 (1-inch) piece fresh ginger, peeled and minced

4 cups Basic Broth (page 59)

1 (8-ounce) package rice noodles

1 bunch chopped fresh spinach

1 tablespoon sesame seeds

Tamari, for seasoning

1. Place the ginger and broth in a large soup pot and bring to a boil.

2. Add the rice noodles and cook for 10 minutes.

3. Stir the spinach into the soup.

4. Remove the pot from the heat, and let stand for 1 minute.

5. Toast the sesame seeds in a dry pan over medium heat for 1 minute.

6. Season the soup with the tamari and serve with a sprinkle of toasted sesame seeds.

⇟ **Ingredient tip** In Autumn, shredded carrots can beautifully replace spinach. Stir the carrots in with the noodles and broth during the last 5 minutes of cooking.

❀ **Season** Year-round. In Summer, it can be made ahead and served at room temperature, spooned over a bowl of fresh greens.

❁ **Dosha** Vata. For Pitta, replace the ginger with ½ teaspoon of Summer Spice Blend (page 61) and serve with fresh mint.

Ginger–Carrot Soup

30 MINUTES OR LESS • KITCHEN REMEDY

Ginger–Carrot Soup is a bowl of radiance, and a warm break from Winter's toll. Its bright orange color offers sunny cheer, not to mention vitamins A, D, and E to strengthen your sight, and selenium to keep your moods sunny and bright. Ayurvedically speaking, it offers sweet, rich, creamy, gingery, hydrating warmth— ideal for Vata days.

SERVES 2

Prep time: 5 minutes

Cook time: 15 minutes

2 tablespoons Ghee (page 58)

1 (1-inch) piece fresh ginger, peeled and roughly chopped

1 teaspoon Autumn Spice Blend (page 62)

6 carrots, chopped

4 cups Basic Broth (page 59)

1 teaspoon lemon zest

Extra-virgin olive oil, for drizzling

2 seasonal herb sprigs, such as thyme, basil, or rosemary, for garnish

1. Melt the ghee in a large soup pot over medium heat. Stir in the ginger and the spice blend, and sauté for 1 minute.

2. Add the carrots and broth and bring to a boil. Reduce the heat to low and simmer for 10 minutes.

3. Transfer the soup to a blender and purée. (Or use an immersion blender or a potato masher for a chunky purée.) Return the soup to the pot and cook for 1 minute more.

4. Serve the soup in bowls sprinkled with the lemon zest, a drizzle of olive oil, and a sprig of seasonal herb.

⇶ **Cooking tip** Thicken the soup by stirring in 1 cup of cubed tofu or sunflower seeds before puréeing, or sweeten it with 1 cup of Homemade Coconut Milk (page 66) stirred in after blending.

✿ **Season** Autumn, Winter

❧ **Dosha** All. Ideal for Vata.

Rice Biryani

Biryani is an Ayurvedic comfort food. Perfect for Autumn, it balances the six tastes with an emphasis on the Vata-reducing properties of sweet. It was originally a Persian dish, so gently tossing the rice with a handful of torn mint leaves before serving keeps with tradition and really brings the dish to life. In Winter, basil is a good alternative to mint.

SERVES 4

Prep time: 5 minutes, plus 30 minutes to soak

Cook time: 25 minutes

1 cup basmati rice

4 tablespoons Ghee (page 58), plus 1 teaspoon

1 tablespoon Seasonal Spice Blend (pages 60–63)

2 cups boiling water

4 small carrots, halved lengthwise and cut into half moons

2 cups finely chopped green beans

½ cup raisins

½ cup cashew pieces

1. Soak the rice for 30 minutes in water. Rinse the rice and set it aside to drain.

2. Melt 4 tablespoons of ghee in a medium pot over medium heat. Add the spice blend and sauté for 1 minute, swirling the pot to combine.

3. Stir in the rice and cook another 2 to 3 minutes, until the ghee is absorbed by the rice.

4. Pour in the water. Cover and bring to a boil, then reduce the heat to low and simmer for 10 minutes.

5. Add the carrots and green beans, and cook for 10 minutes, or until the rice is tender.

6. In a small pan, sauté the raisins and cashews in the remaining 1 teaspoon of ghee until the raisins plump and the cashews are golden.

7. Fluff the rice with a fork. Stir the sautéed raisins and cashews into the pot, and serve warm.

Cooking tip Biryani is a good base for any seasonal vegetables. In addition to carrots and green beans, you can add fresh peas, spinach, chard, kale, celery, zucchini, broccoli, or cauliflower. Toast coconut flakes with the cashews for a tropical sweet crunch. You could also add pistachio, sesame seeds, or chopped olive.

Season Autumn, Winter. For Summer, omit the cashews and use seasonal vegetables.

Dosha With the Autumn Spice Blend (page 62), this is ideal for Vata. For Pitta, use the Summer Spice Blend (page 61) and substitute pumpkin seeds for the cashews. For Kapha, eliminate the cashews and use the Spring Spice Blend (page 60) with a hearty shake of ground ginger or clove, and freshly ground black pepper.

Pho Soup

ONE POT • 30 MINUTES OR LESS • KITCHEN REMEDY

A popular street food in Vietnam, Pho marries the six tastes into one deliciously healthy bowl. Rice noodles or soba, which are made from buckwheat, keep the soup light. Kimchi is a spicy fermented vegetable mix, usually available at grocers in the refrigerated section, but it can be substituted with raw sauerkraut. The point is to get beneficial bacteria that are in fermented vegetables, so look for raw varieties, and don't cook them. Or make your own fermented vegetables by preparing the recipe for Carrot Pickle (page 185).

SERVES 2

Prep time: 5 minutes
Cook time: 5 minutes

2 cups Basic Broth (page 59)

1 head bok choy

2 cups cooked rice noodles

Salt (pink, mineral, or sea), for seasoning

Freshly ground black pepper, for seasoning

1 cup kimchi

2 handfuls mung bean sprouts

1 lime, quartered

1. In a medium soup pot, bring the broth to a boil.

2. Remove the bok choy leaves from the stem. Add the leaves to the broth and cook for 2 minutes.

3. Stir in the noodles and cook for 1 minute.

4. Season with the salt and pepper.

5. Ladle the soup into two bowls.

6. Spoon the kimchi into the bowls and top with the sprouts and lime quarters.

>>> **Serving tip** Divide a cup of cubed tofu between the two bowls, or slice a hardboiled egg lengthwise and lay half in each bowl. Garnish with whole sprigs of basil.

✿ **Season** Year-round

▲ **Dosha** Vata

Curried Green Beans

30 MINUTES OR LESS

Curry is a plant, *and* it is a term for dishes made with various combinations of pungent and healing spices. This recipe enhances the heat of the Winter Spice Blend (page 63) with fresh ginger to create a light supper, and also pairs perfectly with rice or soba noodles for heartier meals. Hazelnuts have a strong nutty taste and a spectrum of health benefits, including the healthy fat that can be so crucial for Vata.

SERVES 2

Prep time: 5 minutes
Cook time: 10 minutes

1 teaspoon salt, plus additional for seasoning

1 pound green beans, cut into ½-inch pieces

2 tablespoons Ghee (page 58), divided

½ teaspoon brown mustard seeds

1 (½-inch) piece fresh ginger, minced

½ teaspoon Winter Spice Blend (page 63)

½ cup hazelnuts, coarsely chopped

1 teaspoon tamari

Freshly ground black pepper, for seasoning

1 bunch chopped flat-leaf parsley

1. Bring a pot of water to a boil. Add 1 teaspoon of salt. Fill a large bowl with water and ice.

2. Add the green beans to the boiling water and cook for 2 minutes.

3. Drain the beans and immediately immerse them in the ice water. When completely cool, drain the beans and lay them on towels to dry.

4. Melt 1 tablespoon of ghee in a medium saucepan over medium-high heat. Add the mustard seeds. As soon as they begin to pop, stir in the ginger and the spice blend. Reduce the heat to medium, cover the pan, and cook for 1 minute.

5. Add the green beans and stir to coat them in the spicy ghee. Cover the pan and cook for 5 minutes.

6. In a small pan, melt the remaining 1 tablespoon of ghee over medium heat. Add the hazelnuts and toast them until they are golden, stirring frequently. Remove the pan from the heat.

7. Once the beans are tender-crisp, remove the pan from the heat. Stir in the tamari. Season with salt and pepper. Toss with the hazelnuts, and top with the parsley.

>>> **Serving tip** Serve over Rice Biryani (page 132) with fresh basil and lime juice.

Season Autumn, Winter, Spring

Dosha Vata. For Pitta, Kapha, replace the cashews with pumpkin seeds.

Borscht

Borscht is Eastern European soul food, with colorful roots that hold their vitality, and fermented vegetables that feed digestion, and the ideal warmth for the dark, cold days of Winter. Alternating tastes of sweet and sour to produce a light meal with deep flavor, this rich ruby soup is a Winter gem. Traditional recipes call for sauerkraut to be cooked into the soup. Instead, add the sauerkraut after ladling the soup into bowls to preserve the healthy benefits of that good fermentation.

SERVES 4

Prep time: 10 minutes

Cook time: 1 hour

4 beets

1 small sweet potato

1 tablespoon Ghee (page 58), plus 1 teaspoon

1 (½-inch) piece fresh ginger, minced

1 teaspoon Winter Spice Blend (page 63)

4 cups Basic Broth (page 59)

Salt (pink, mineral, or sea), for seasoning

Freshly ground black pepper, for seasoning

½ cup sauerkraut with juices

1. Preheat the oven to 450°F. Line a baking sheet with parchment paper.

2. Scrub the beets and sweet potato, trimming away the beet greens but keeping the stems, tops, and tails intact to hold in the juices while they roast. Pierce the sweet potato with a fork to create steam holes.

3. Rub the beets and sweet potato with 1 teaspoon of ghee and sprinkle with the salt. Place on the baking sheet and roast for about 45 minutes, or until a knife slides easily through the center. Let cool, then peel and cut into bite-size pieces.

4. Melt the remaining 1 tablespoon of ghee in a large pot over medium heat. Stir in the ginger and the spice blend and swirl to stir.

5. Add the beets, sweet potato, and broth, and bring to a boil. Reduce the heat to low and simmer for 10 minutes.

6. Transfer about one-quarter of the soup to a blender and lightly purée it to make it creamy-chunky. Stir this back into the pot and warm for 1 minute more.

7. Remove the pot from the heat and let cool for 3 minutes. Season with salt and pepper.

8. Divide the soup between bowls and serve with a generous spoonful of sauerkraut.

>>> **Serving tip** Serve with a dollop of yogurt, a sprig of dill, and a warm chapati.

⚙ **Season** Autumn, Winter. For Summer, forgo the sauerkraut and simmer with fresh cabbage.

◬ **Dosha** Vata. Good for Pitta with Summer Spice Blend (page 61); omit the ginger and substitute fresh shredded cabbage for the sauerkraut.

Fennel & Fava Bean Soup

ONE POT

Also known as broad beans, fava beans are a great source of lean protein and fiber. In Spring, fresh favas are delicious fresh from the pod and tossed with salads. Once dried, they require a good soaking, but after cooking they become soft, creamy, and sweet—well worth the wait. Sometimes I make this more as a mash, like refried beans, by adjusting how much broth gets added back. Either way, this recipe is a delicious gift from Sicily, where it has been traditional farm fare since ancient times.

SERVES 4

Prep time: 15 minutes, plus 12 hours to soak

Cook time: 1½ hours

2 cups dried fava beans

4 cups Basic Broth (page 59)

4 cups water

1 lemon

1 fennel bulb and feathery fronds, chopped

2 celery stalks, chopped

2 tablespoons Ghee (page 58)

1 teaspoon sea salt, plus additional for seasoning

Freshly ground black pepper, for seasoning

Extra-virgin olive oil, for drizzling

4 fresh oregano sprigs or mint leaves, for garnish

1. Place the beans in a large bowl and cover with cold water by several inches. Soak for 12 hours.

2. Drain the beans and rinse them well. Put them in a large soup pot with the broth and water. Bring to a boil on medium-high heat, then reduce heat to medium-low. Cover and simmer for 1 hour, until the beans open and start to come apart.

3. Zest and juice the lemon. Reserve 1 teaspoon of zest for garnish.

4. Stir in the fennel bulb, fennel fronds, and celery with the beans and simmer for another 30 minutes, or until the beans are very tender.

5. Drain the beans, reserving the broth. Remove the large fronds and discard. Transfer the beans to a bowl.

6. In the same soup pot, heat the ghee over medium-low heat.

7. Put the beans and fennel in a blender with the salt and 1 cup of the reserved broth, and purée, then pour the mixture back into the soup pot. Stir in more broth, 1 cup at a time, until you have the consistency you desire.

8. Stir in the lemon juice and zest. Heat for another 1 or 2 minutes to ensure the soup is very hot.

9. Taste and season with salt and pepper. Serve with a drizzle of olive oil, a garnish of lemon zest, and a sprig of oregano or a few leaves of fresh mint.

Recipe tip Like lentils and chickpeas, fava beans have been a part of eastern Mediterranean cooking for eons, and like their legume cousins, they can be prepared in myriad ways. For extra nutrients and flavor, stir in a couple of chopped carrots or a bunch of chopped dandelion leaves at the time you add the fennel. Experiment with dried Mediterranean herbs, curry powder, ground chipotle, or fresh herbs to find the flavor highlights you like best. With dried herbs, sauté them with the ghee just before adding the cooked beans back into the pot. With fresh herbs, float them on the soup when serving.

Season Autumn, Winter, Spring

Dosha All

Seasonal Vegetable Purée

30 MINUTES OR LESS

This is quick and easy to make. The prep is just a quick chop of veggies and then cook, purée, and serve. Since it is a blended soup, chopping the vegetables can be quick and rough. Look for a variety of colors and textures in your seasonal vegetables—turnips, beets, daikon radishes, cauliflower, fresh peas, purple carrots, and asparagus.

SERVES 2

Prep time: 5 minutes

Cook time: 15 minutes

2 cups roughly chopped seasonal vegetables

1 cup Basic Broth (page 59)

1 teaspoon Seasonal Spice Blend (pages 60–63)

1 (1-inch) strip kombu

1 cup chopped leafy greens, such as spinach, kale, collards, dandelion leaves, or chard

Salt (pink, mineral, or sea), for seasoning

Freshly ground black pepper, for seasoning

1. Put the vegetables, broth, spice blend, and kombu in a medium pot and bring to a boil.

2. Cook for 10 minutes, then add the leafy greens and cook for 2 minutes more.

3. Purée the vegetables with an immersion blender, or transfer them to a blender to purée.

4. Season with salt and pepper, and serve.

⋙ **Serving tip** Garnish each bowl with a sprig of fresh rosemary for Autumnal beauty. In Spring, garnish with basil, in Summer with dill or cilantro, in Winter with a whole leaf of sage. Or top with a generous dollop of Cilantro Pesto (page 174) or Basil Pesto (page 175) for bigger flavor.

❀ **Season** Year-round. In Summer, allow the purée to cool almost to room temperature before serving.

△ **Dosha** All

Healing Kanji

ONE POT • KITCHEN REMEDY

Kanji is an ideal healing soup for its mild tasting, highly nutritious, easily digestible warmth, and is especially good for upset stomach or debilitation. In the southern Indian state of Kerala, kanji is eaten primarily for breakfast or supper. It can also substitute for rice to accompany mung dal or steamed vegetables, or simply be stirred into a curry. The strained rice water is great in dal, stews, soups; use instead of water for creamier broth. The strained rice can be served with sautéed vegetables, or tossed into a salad, like Pistachio Rice with Tahini Yogurt (page 113).

SERVES 4

Prep time: 5 minutes

Cook time: 1 hour

½ cup basmati rice

6 cups water

1 tablespoon Ghee (page 58)

1 teaspoon salt
(pink, mineral, or sea)

Freshly ground black pepper

1. Put the rice in the center of a kitchen towel. Draw the ends of the towel together and twist to get a ball of rice. Bang the rice against the counter to "break" it.

2. Rinse the rice under cool water and place it in a large pot with the water.

3. Bring to a boil, then reduce the heat to very low. Cover the pot and simmer for 1 hour.

4. Stir in the ghee and season with the salt and pepper.

➤➤ **Cooking tip** For a creamier, slightly sweeter version, replace 1 cup of water with 1 cup of dairy or Homemade Coconut Milk (page 66). For a more savory version, use equal parts vegetable broth and water.

✿ **Season** Year-round

◓ **Dosha** Vata, Pitta

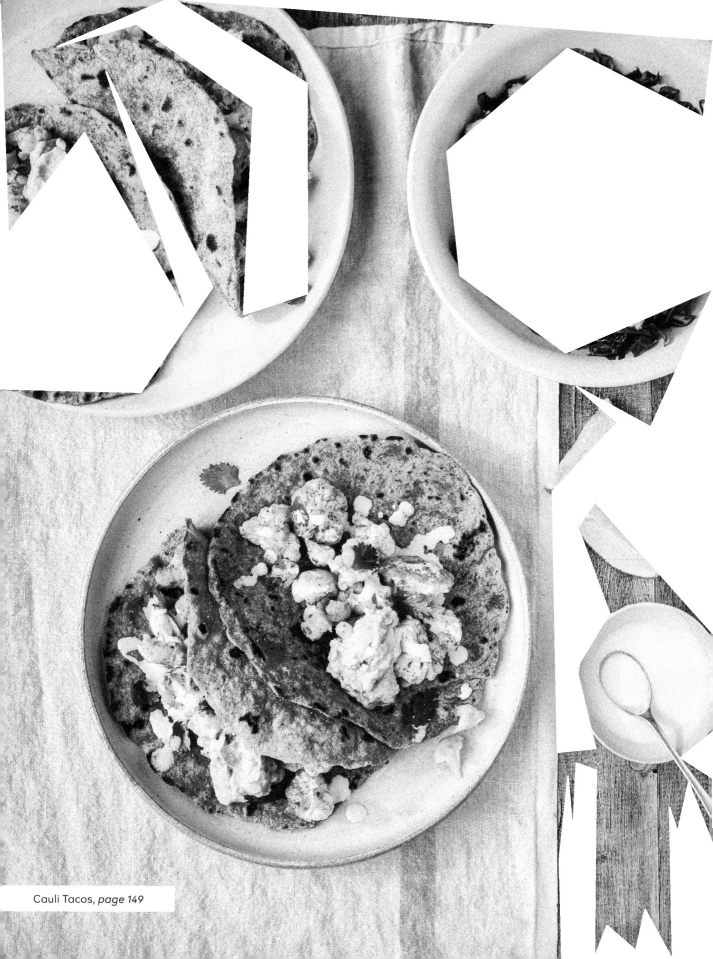

Cauli Tacos, *page 149*

nine

Ayurvedic Spins on Favorites

Kitchari "Burgers" 144

Pasta al Pesto 145

Lentil Lasagna 146

Rice & Bean Burritos 148

Cauli Tacos 149

Yam Fries 150

Flatbread Pizza 151

Quesadillas 152

Gravy & Mash 153

Whole-Skillet Hash Browns 154

PLT Sandwiches 156

Sweet Potato Jackets 157

Kitchari "Burgers"

30 MINUTES OR LESS • KITCHEN REMEDY

I am often asked how to make Ayurvedic meals appealing to the whole family. Since kitchari is such an Ayurvedic staple, I've looked for a number of ways over the years to make it appealing to all. This recipe is popular with Ayurveda beginners and longtime practitioners as a quick and fun way to serve it to children. Nutritional yeast is optional, but it does lend a cheesy taste and B vitamins. If you eat eggs, beat 1 egg and lightly stir it in with the kitchari before it rests. Although strictly speaking Ayurveda does not like us to mix our proteins, it will give your burger better hold and a crisper golden edge.

SERVES 4

Prep time: 15 minutes
Cook time: 20 minutes

2 cups Kitchari (Spring, Summer, Autumn, or Winter; use what's in season)

2 tablespoons psyllium husks

1 tablespoon nutritional yeast (optional)

1 tablespoon Ghee (page 58)

½ teaspoon ground ginger

¼ teaspoon salt (pink, mineral, or sea)

1. Put the kitchari in a medium bowl and stir in the psyllium and nutritional yeast (if using) to mix well, ideally with your hands. Let the mixture sit for 10 minutes at room temperature.

2. Melt the ghee in a saucepan over medium-high heat. Sprinkle in the ginger and salt, and swirl the pan to combine.

3. Take a small handful of the kitchari mixture, form it into a ball, then press to flatten it into a burger. Put the burger in the pan and cook until it browns, about 5 minutes. Flip and cover the pan while the burger browns on the second side, about 5 minutes more. Repeat until all the kitchari batter is used.

4. Keep the patties warm in the oven on low heat until you're ready to serve. Or make smaller patties and serve them at a party as sliders.

⇢))⸱ **Serving tip** Serve with Yogurt-Dill Dipping Sauce (page 182) and cucumbers, on a toasted bun, or over a salad.

✿ **Season** Year-round

◭ **Dosha** All

Pasta al Pesto

ONE POT • **30 MINUTES OR LESS**

This classic from the Italian Riviera includes basil, which is balancing for Vata and Kapha, and in smaller amounts, good for Pitta, too. A warming herb, basil lends sweet, pungent, and bitter tastes. This dish also has spinach for astringency and lemon to round out the six tastes.

SERVES 4

Prep time: 5 minutes

Cook time: 15 minutes

1 (8-ounce) package rice noodles

2 cups chopped fresh spinach

1 cup Basil Pesto (page 175)

1 teaspoon extra-virgin olive oil

1 tablespoon lemon zest

Salt (pink, mineral, or sea), for seasoning

Freshly ground black pepper, for seasoning

Fresh basil, for garnish

1. Cook the noodles according to the package instructions. Drain, reserving ½ cup of the pasta water.

2. Put the pot back on the stove over medium heat and add the reserved pasta water and spinach. Cook for 3 minutes.

3. Stir in the noodles. Spoon in the pesto, olive oil, and lemon zest and toss.

4. Season with salt and pepper.

5. Serve garnished with fresh basil.

⇉ **Serving tip** Sprinkle with red pepper flakes in Winter and Spring.

❀ **Season** Year-round

⬥ **Dosha** All

Lentil Lasagna

In this vegan twist on lasagna, ribbons of zucchini stand in for pasta, lentils and sun-dried tomatoes replace ground meat, and a nutty pesto bakes it up golden and rich. If you have trouble digesting lentils, try cooking with kombu, an edible seaweed that neutralizes the gas-producing compounds in beans. (Cut a 1-inch strip of kombu and boil it with the lentils.) The Autumn or Winter seasonal spice blends are best with this dish.

SERVES 4

Prep time: 20 minutes, plus overnight to soak

Cook time: 40 minutes

1 cup lentils

1 lemon wedge

2 shallots, diced

¼ cup sun-dried tomatoes, packed in oil

3 cups water, plus more as needed

Salt (pink, mineral, or sea)

1 tablespoon Ghee (page 58)

1 teaspoon Seasonal Spice Blend (pages 60–63)

3 medium zucchini, thinly sliced lengthwise

1 cup Basil Pesto (page 175) made with ½ cup pine nuts

Freshly ground black pepper, for seasoning

1. Rinse the lentils under cool water and put in a medium bowl. Cover with boiled water and a squeeze of lemon juice. Soak overnight at room temperature.

2. Chop the shallots and drain the lentils.

3. Transfer the lentils to a large pot along with the shallots and sun-dried tomatoes. Add the water, enough to cover the ingredients.

4. Bring to a boil, then reduce the heat to low and simmer for 20 minutes, or until the lentils are soft. Stir in a few pinches of salt, and remove the pot from the heat.

5. Preheat the oven to 350°F.

6. Melt the ghee in a medium saucepan over medium heat. Stir in the spice blend and sauté for 1 minute.

7. Increase the heat to medium-high, and add the zucchini slices in a single layer (working in batches if necessary) and cook for 2 minutes. Turn the slices over and cook for 3 minutes more or until the zucchini start to brown.

8. Spoon the cooked lentils into an 8-by-8-inch casserole dish and spread evenly. Layer the zucchini slices on top of the lentils. Spoon the pesto over the zucchini, spreading it evenly over the entire top layer. Season with the salt and pepper.

9. Bake for 12 minutes, or until the pine nuts in the pesto turn golden brown.

≫ **Substitution tip** Pine nuts bake up to give a cheesy flavor to this dish, but walnuts are a good replacement if pine nuts are hard to find or too expensive.

✿ **Season** Autumn, Winter

❀ **Dosha** All

Rice & Bean Burritos

30 MINUTES OR LESS

Kitchari is so beneficial and so healing that we want everyone to enjoy it. Sometimes, though, it takes a little creativity to get our picky eaters to try it. This dish is a great way to use up what's left over from lunch and to share your favorite kitchari recipe with family or friends at dinner. You don't even have to tell them how good it is for them.

SERVES 2

Prep time: 15 minutes

Cook time: 15 minutes

1 handful cherry tomatoes, halved or quartered

1 teaspoon freshly squeezed lime juice

Salt (pink, mineral, or sea), for seasoning

Freshly ground black pepper, for seasoning

2 (8-inch or 12-inch) whole-wheat tortillas

1 cup Kitchari (Spring, Summer, Autumn, or Winter)

½ avocado, sliced

2 tablespoons Cucumber Raita (page 180)

1. Preheat the oven to its lowest setting.

2. Put the tomatoes in a small bowl, drizzle with the lime juice, and season with salt and pepper. Let sit for at least 10 minutes, stirring occasionally.

3. Heat your oven to its lowest setting. Stack the tortillas on a baking sheet and warm them in the oven for 5 to 10 minutes.

4. Warm the kitchari to piping hot in a small saucepan over medium-high heat.

5. Assemble the burritos: Spoon half the kitchari in a line down the middle of a tortilla. Layer slices of avocado on top. Nestle a spoonful of tomatoes alongside the kitchari. Drizzle 1 tablespoon of raita over the top. Fold up the bottom of the tortilla, then fold in the two sides. Roll the burrito and squeeze while doing so to tighten the fold. Repeat for the second burrito.

>>> **Serving tip** Garnish with cilantro and a wedge of lime. Serve with Spring Pea Salad (page 102) or Persian Cucumber Salad (page 105), or with steamed greens. Use plain yogurt if a raita substitute is needed. Substitute chopped cucumber for tomatoes.

✿ **Season** Year-round

❀ **Dosha** All

Cauli Tacos

30 MINUTES OR LESS

In Southern California, Baja tacos are on almost every menu, with restaurants competing to serve the best. Using cauliflower, you can make a vegetarian version every bit as tasty—while supportive to all three doshas. For a crowd-pleasing "Baja" crunch, while the cauliflower is still damp from rinsing, roll the florets in rice, almond, or coconut flour and then sauté. Let your children and friends help you create these fun tacos for lunch, dinner, or parties.

MAKES 4 TACOS

Prep time: 5 minutes
Cook time: 10 minutes

3 tablespoons Ghee (page 58)

1 head cauliflower, cut into bite-size florets

Salt (pink, mineral, or sea), for seasoning

Freshly ground black pepper, for seasoning

½ teaspoon paprika

¼ cup mayonnaise

Juice of ½ lime

1 tablespoon brine from Carrot Pickle (page 185), or any pickle juice

4 Chapatis (page 69; double the recipe)

Avocado Mash (page 184)

1. Melt the ghee in a large skillet over medium heat. Once sizzling hot, add the cauliflower. Cook for 8 minutes, until golden, stirring occasionally.

2. Use a slotted spoon to transfer the florets to a paper towel–lined plate. Season with salt, pepper, and the paprika.

3. In a small bowl, whisk together the mayonnaise, lime juice, and brine to make a white sauce.

4. Assemble the tacos: Spoon some cauliflower onto the center of a chapati and add a dollop of avocado mash. Drizzle with the white sauce. Repeat to make the rest of the tacos, and serve.

>>> **Serving tip** Garnish with lime wedges and cilantro. Pair with Mango & Cabbage Salad (page 106).

❀ **Season** Summer, Autumn

◭ **Dosha** Vata, Pitta

Yam Fries

Making Ayurvedic cooking appeal to the whole family can be a challenge, but these warm, grounding, and nutritious yam fries delight everyone, especially kids. Sweet, dense, and heavy, they are nonetheless *sattvic* and ideal for all doshas, even Kapha when you double the dose of spices. Your Spring spice blend is excellent here, but so is a curry powder, ground chipotle powder, cinnamon, or any of your favorite spices. Enjoy the yam fries as an afternoon snack, or serve them with Kitchari "Burgers" (page 144) for an Ayurvedic twist on a favorite American meal.

SERVES 2

Prep time: 5 minutes, plus 1 hour to soak

Cook time: 30 minutes

1 yam

1 tablespoon coconut oil

1 tablespoon Spring Spice Blend (page 60)

2 teaspoons cornstarch

1 tablespoon salt (pink, mineral, or sea)

1. Scrub the yam and cut it into ¼-inch-thick fries. Place in a bowl with cold water and soak for 1 hour. Strain and set on a kitchen towel to dry thoroughly.

2. Preheat the oven to 425°F and position a rack in the center of the oven. Line a baking sheet with parchment paper.

3. Melt the coconut oil in a medium skillet over medium heat. Add the spice blend and swirl to combine. Remove from the heat.

4. Put the yam fries in a bowl or a large zip-top bag and toss with the cornstarch. Pour the spicy oil over and give them another good shake.

5. Set the fries in a single layer on the prepared baking sheet, being careful not to overcrowd. Bake for 15 minutes, flip the fries, again spreading them evenly so they don't touch. Bake for another 10 to 15 minutes, or until browned.

6. Turn the oven off, open the door slightly, and let the fries sit for 10 minutes to release steam and cool.

7. Toss the fries with the salt as soon as they come out of the oven, and enjoy warm.

⫸ **Cooking tip** Spread the fries evenly on the baking sheet; don't let them touch. Open the oven door a couple of times during cooking to release steam.

❀ **Season** Summer, Autumn, Winter

🜂 **Dosha** Vata, Pitta

Flatbread Pizza

30 MINUTES OR LESS

Homemade pizza can be a great way to encourage children to eat healthy. Ask for their help in making the chapatis and assembling the pizzas. Let them add their favorite vegetables in addition to the zucchini. They will enjoy it even more if they are invested in the creativity. This flatbread is also delicious when served with Yogurt-Dill Dipping Sauce (page 182).

MAKES 2 SMALL PIZZAS

Prep time: 5 minutes
Cook time: 15 minutes

1 teaspoon Ghee (page 58)

½ teaspoon Seasonal Spice Blend (pages 60–63)

1 zucchini, thinly sliced

2 Chapatis (page 69)

½ cup Basil Pesto (page 175) or Cilantro Pesto (page 174)

½ cup Paneer (page 100)

1. Preheat the oven to 350°F.

2. Melt the ghee in a saucepan over medium heat. Add the spice blend and swirl the pan to combine. Add the zucchini and sauté for 3 minutes. Transfer the zucchini to a plate with a slotted spoon.

3. Put the chapatis on a baking sheet. Pour the ghee used to sauté the zucchini over each chapati.

4. Spread the pesto across the chapatis. Layer on the zucchini. Crumble the paneer and sprinkle it evenly over the zucchini.

5. Bake for 10 minutes, or until the edges of the chapati begin to brown and the topping bubbles. Let cool for a few minutes before serving.

Ingredient tip Zucchini gets soggy if cooked too long, so sauté it just until translucent.

Season Year-round

Dosha All. For Pitta, replace the Basil Pesto with Cilantro Pesto (page 174). For Kapha, sprinkle with red pepper flakes or cayenne.

Quesadillas

Lighter than traditional quesadillas and less oily, these quesadillas are still rich and delicious. Serve with a big bowl of Avocado Mash (page 184) and they will become a family favorite.

SERVES 2

Prep time: 5 minutes
Cook time: 10 minutes

¼ cup Paneer (page 100)

2 teaspoons Ghee (page 58), divided

Salt (pink, mineral, or sea), for seasoning

Freshly ground black pepper, for seasoning

2 large Chapatis (page 69)

1. In a small bowl, mash the paneer. Add 1 teaspoon of ghee and stir until creamy. Season with the salt and pepper.

2. Melt the remaining 1 teaspoon of ghee in a skillet over medium heat. Put a chapati in the pan. Spoon half the paneer across half the chapati. With a spatula, fold the chapati in half to cover the paneer, and press down. Cook for 2 minutes. Flip and cook for 3 minutes more, or until the chapati is lightly browned on both sides. Repeat with the second chapati.

≫ **Serving tip** Enjoy with a salad for lunch or with steamed greens for dinner.

✿ **Season** Summer, Autumn, Winter

🔻 **Dosha** Vata, Pitta

Gravy & Mash

ONE POT · 30 MINUTES OR LESS

While onions and garlic are considered *rajasic*, used sparingly they can be medicinal, helping ward off winter colds. This vegetarian gravy is a sweet comfort that can be served over mash as here, or spooned into a Sweet Potato Jacket (page 157), poured over Roasted Roots Ecrasse (page 129), or used as a dipping sauce for Chapatis (page 69). It is a perfect gravy for holiday meals.

MAKES 2 CUPS

Prep time: 10 minutes

Cook time: 20 minutes

½ cup Ghee (page 58)

¼ cup chopped shallots

2 garlic cloves, minced

½ cup whole-wheat flour

¼ cup tamari

2 cups Basic Broth (page 59)

½ teaspoon dried sage

Salt (pink, mineral, or sea), for seasoning

Freshly ground black pepper, for seasoning

Sweet Potato Jackets (page 157), peeled and mashed

1. Melt the ghee in a medium saucepan over medium heat. Add the shallots and garlic, and sauté until soft and translucent, about 5 minutes.

2. Stir in the flour and tamari to form a smooth paste. Gradually whisk in the broth. Stir in the sage, and season with salt and pepper.

3. Bring to a gentle boil, then reduce the heat to low and simmer, stirring constantly, for 8 to 10 minutes, or until thickened.

4. Ladle some of the gravy over the roasted sweet potatoes.

⇢⇢ **Ingredient tip** Wheat flour has gluten, which helps this gravy bind and thicken. If you use a gluten-free flour, choose a flour combined with starches so the gravy will congeal.

✿ **Season** Autumn, Winter

◬ **Dosha** Vata

Whole-Skillet Hash Browns

Hash browns are a healthy breakfast choice when, as here, they are made from sweet potatoes, and combined with flaxseed, orange juice, and coconut oil. Low in fat yet rich in taste, sweet potatoes are a more nutritious, sumptuous, and colorful choice than regular potatoes. Soaking the sweet potato prior to cooking draws out the starch and helps the hash brown up. Enjoy this on its own or with a side of eggs, beans, or even a seasonal kitchari. It also makes a great snack and an easy dinner when served with a side of sautéed greens.

SERVES 4

Prep time: 10 minutes, plus 1 hour to soak

Cook time: 30 minutes

1 sweet potato, grated

Salt (pink, mineral, or sea)

1 tablespoon flaxseed, ground

1 teaspoon chia seeds

1 orange

1 teaspoon Seasonal Spice Blend (pages 60–63)

Freshly ground black pepper

2 tablespoons coconut oil, divided

1. Put the grated sweet potato in a large bowl and fill the bowl with cold water and a pinch of salt. Soak for 1 hour. Drain and set on a kitchen towel, and pat dry.

2. Meanwhile, grate the orange peel to make 1 teaspoon zest, and squeeze ¼ cup of orange juice.

3. In a medium bowl, mix the sweet potato with the ground flaxseed, chia seeds, orange zest, orange juice, and spice blend. Sprinkle with salt and pepper. Let stand for 10 minutes.

4. Melt 1 tablespoon of coconut oil in a medium skillet over medium heat. Spoon in the sweet potato mixture. Using the back of the spoon, spread evenly across the skillet. Cook uncovered for 10 minutes, then cover and cook for another 10 minutes.

5. To brown the other side, you have two choices: One way is to set your oven to broil, uncover the skillet, and place it on the top shelf of the oven for 10 minutes, watching to be sure it doesn't burn. The other way is to uncover the pan, hold a plate over the hash, and flip the pan over to turn the hash onto the plate, and slide the hash from the plate back into the pan. Cook uncovered on medium heat for another 10 minutes.

6. Meanwhile, in a small saucepan, melt the remaining 1 tablespoon of coconut oil. When the hash browns are done, slide them onto a serving plate and drizzle with the coconut oil. Taste and season with another pinch of salt and another grind of black pepper if needed.

>>> **Serving tip** Serve with a dollop of yogurt or a smear of paneer, with a fried egg, or with Seasonal Fruit Compote (page 89) for a makeshift pancake.

✿ **Season** Year-round

◈ **Dosha** All

PLT Sandwiches

Most of the world does not eat sandwiches for lunch, and sandwiches certainly aren't included in traditional Ayurvedic fare. Still, a sandwich is sometimes the very best thing—for picnics, school lunches, working meals, and travel sustenance. This unique pumpkin seed, lettuce, and tomato sandwich features a minty mayo with a light, crunchy texture that comes from toasting the coconut and the pumpkin seeds. It's almost like a BLT, but better.

MAKES 2 SANDWICHES

Prep time: 5 minutes

Cook time: 5 minutes

1 tomato, cut into slices

Salt (pink, mineral, or sea), for seasoning

Freshly ground black pepper, for seasoning

¼ cup raw pumpkin seeds

¼ cup coconut flakes

1 teaspoon Ghee (page 58)

1 teaspoon tamari

2 tablespoons mayonnaise, plus 2 teaspoons

1 large handful fresh mint leaves

4 slices whole-grain bread, toasted

4 red leaf lettuce leaves

1. Place the tomato slices on a plate and season with salt and pepper.

2. Toast the pumpkin seeds and coconut flakes in a small pan over a medium-high heat. After 2 minutes, add the ghee. Swirl the pan to stir, and toast for 2 minutes more.

3. When the flakes start to lightly brown, turn off the heat, add the tamari, and swirl again.

4. Transfer the pumpkin seeds and coconut flakes to a small bowl and stir in 2 tablespoons of mayonnaise. Tear the mint leaves into strips and stir them into the bowl.

5. Spoon a generous layer of minty mayo on 2 slices of the bread. Spread the remaining 2 teaspoons of mayonnaise across the other 2 slices. Layer the tomatoes over the minty mayo, and lettuce leaves over the tomatoes. Top the sandwiches with the mayonnaise-dressed 2 slices of bread. Gently press to close, and serve.

>>> **Serving tip** This is every bit as good without toasting the bread, and is excellent with Avocado Mash (page 184) or avocado slices. Layer in grilled zucchini, slices of roasted squash, fresh cucumber, or your favorite sandwich fillings.

✿ **Season** Summer

🌰 **Dosha** Pitta. For Vata, drain a spoonful of sauerkraut and layer it into the sandwich for something close to a veg Reuben.

Sweet Potato Jackets

Sometimes the best meals are the simplest. Scrub a tater, pop it in the oven, slice it open, slather it with ghee, and you have divine deliciousness. In London, where I lived in my early adult life, street vendors sell baked potatoes stuffed with your choice of a great variety of fillings to make a meal. There they call them "jackets." Swap a white potato with a sweet potato, and you have a healthy alternative to this easy comfort food.

SERVES 2

Prep time: 5 minutes
Cook time: 45 minutes

1 tablespoon Ghee (page 58), plus more for serving

Salt (pink, mineral, or sea), for seasoning

1 teaspoon Seasonal Spice Blend (pages 60–63)

2 sweet potatoes, scrubbed well

Freshly ground black pepper, for seasoning

¼ cup plain whole yogurt

2 tablespoons chopped dill

1. Preheat the oven to 475°F.

2. Line a baking sheet with parchment paper and spoon the ghee into the middle. Place the baking sheet in the oven to melt the ghee.

3. Sprinkle the melted ghee with the spice blend and a few pinches of salt. Roll the sweet potatoes in the ghee.

4. Roast the sweet potatoes for 45 minutes, or until a knife slides easily through the centers.

5. Let cool a few minutes, then slice lengthwise, lather with more ghee, and season with salt and pepper. Spoon the yogurt into the center of each sweet potato and sprinkle with the dill.

➢➢ **Serving tip** For Vata, use Tahini Yogurt (page 113). For Pitta, substitute the yogurt with Simple Saag (page 124). For Kapha, serve with Basil Pesto (page 175). For family meals, spoon in Delicious Dal (page 115) before adding a topping of yogurt.

✿ **Season** Autumn

◭ **Dosha** Vata, Pitta

Nutty-Crusted Apple Pie, *page 166*

ten
Soothing Savories & Sweets

Apricot Tapioca Pudding 160

Curried Cashews 161

Spicy Popcorn 162

Stuffed Dates 163

Pistachio Truffles 164

Chocolate Pudding 165

Nutty-Crusted Apple Pie 166

Carrot Halva 168

Coconut-Mango Crumble 169

Healthy Hot Chocolate 170

Easy Homemade Jam 171

Apricot Tapioca Pudding

30 MINUTES OR LESS

My mother was the master in the kitchen, and gave us a refined appreciation for the art of life, but on weekends, Dad was the playful food explorer. On country drives, he would always stop at roadside farm stands—excitedly buying more than we could ever eat. On Saturdays, he'd gather us children to help make pancakes, fresh bread, ice cream, and for one brief period, tapioca. In those days, tapioca meant time with Dad. Now it is a taste reminder of a father's love. It is a throwback that meets modern requirements—a clean, light, grain-free, dairy-free dessert that doubles as a warm, sweet breakfast. It is excellent for Kapha, and perfect in the Spring paired with the season's stone fruits like plums, peaches, or in this case apricots.

SERVES 2

Prep time: 5 minutes

Cook time: 20 minutes

1¾ cups water, divided

½ cup tapioca pearls

1 teaspoon Ghee (page 58)

½ teaspoon ground cinnamon

¼ teaspoon ground ginger

Pinch salt (pink, mineral, or sea)

12 dried apricots, roughly chopped

1 cup plain yogurt

2 tablespoons honey

½ teaspoon lemon zest

1. Bring 1½ cups of water to a boil in a small saucepan. Stir in the tapioca pearls. Return the water to a boil, cover the pan, and reduce the heat to low. Simmer the tapioca for about 10 minutes. It is done when the pearls have dissolved and the tapioca is creamy.

2. Melt the ghee in a saucepan on medium-low heat. Stir in the cinnamon, ginger, and salt, and sauté for 1 minute. Add the apricots and stir to coat them with the spicy ghee. Increase the heat to medium-high and add the remaining ¼ cup of water. Bring to a boil, then remove the pan from the heat. Let the apricots sit for about 5 minutes.

3. Transfer the apricots and liquid to a blender. Pulse a few times to mince the apricots, keeping a chunky consistency. Spoon the tapioca into a serving bowl. Swirl in the yogurt and the apricot mixture. Drizzle with the honey and sprinkle with the lemon zest.

>>> **Serving tip** Garnish with mint for a bright pop of flavor.

⚙ **Season** Spring

🜂 **Dosha** Kapha

Curried Cashews

30 MINUTES OR LESS

Surprisingly, there are no ground curry leaves in curry powder, which is simply a mixture of sweet and pungent ground spices originally called curry by the British during their occupation of India. Curry leaves aren't even spicy or pungent. Like a smaller, shinier bay leaf and just as excellent an ingredient to use in cooking legumes, curry leaves are ubiquitous in South Indian cooking, where they are prized for their citrusy aroma and Ayurvedic benefits. You can usually find them at Asian grocers or you can buy them fresh online. They make all the difference in this recipe, but in a pinch can be substituted with basil leaves.

MAKES 1 CUP

Prep time: 5 minutes

Cook time: 10 minutes

1 teaspoon coconut oil

Pinch mustard seeds

1 cup raw cashews

1 teaspoon Seasonal Spice Blend (pages 60–63)

1 handful curry leaves

Salt (pink, mineral, or sea), for seasoning

1. Melt the oil in a saucepan over a medium heat. Add the mustard seeds and sauté just until they pop.

2. Stir in the cashews, spice blend, and curry leaves. Toast for 5 minutes, stirring occasionally, until the cashews begin to brown.

3. Remove the pan from the heat. Season with a generous amount of salt. Taste and adjust the seasonings as needed.

4. Let the cashews cool in the pan for about 3 minutes, then transfer them to a serving bowl.

5. Store in an airtight glass jar at room temperature.

⇥ **Storage tip** The cashews are good for about 1 week and are best slightly warm.

✿ **Season** Autumn

◭ **Dosha** Vata

Spicy Popcorn

30 MINUTES OR LESS

Craving crunch might be your body's way of trying to balance Kapha, and this is that perfect Kapha treat. It has the light, dry, and hot qualities of popcorn, pungent spices that act as diuretics to help reduce Kapha's tendency toward water retention, and is creamy and delicious, but lighter than butter ghee.

MAKES 1 CUP

Prep time: 5 minutes

Cook time: 5 minutes

1 tablespoon coconut oil

¼ cup organic
popcorn kernels

1 tablespoon Ghee (page 58)

1 teaspoon Spring Spice
Blend (page 60)

1. Melt the oil in a large soup pot over medium heat. Toss in 1 kernel and cover the pot with a lid. When the kernel pops, toss in the rest of the kernels. Shake the pot while the kernels heat and pop, lifting the lid slightly about every 30 seconds to release steam. Once the kernels are popped, transfer the popcorn to a large serving bowl.

2. In a small saucepan, melt the ghee over medium heat. Stir in the spice blend and swirl the pan to combine.

3. Drizzle the popcorn with the curried ghee and toss to combine.

Ingredient tip While corn is a heating grain, when popped it is light, dry, and rough, so Vata people really should avoid it. Be sure to use organic kernels.

Season Late Winter, Spring

Dosha Kapha

Stuffed Dates

30 MINUTES OR LESS

Dates are sweet, *sattvic*, and *ojas* enhancing, nourishing reproductive tissue and the immune system. Almonds, too, are considered a great *rasayana*, or rejuvenative, making this a deeply tonifying treat for Vata. Rich and grounding, Stuffed Dates make a great after-school snack for children. They are also delicious when sliced and served in a warm bowl of breakfast porridge.

MAKES 8

Prep time: 5 minutes

8 Medjool dates

4 teaspoons almond butter

Autumn Spice Blend (page 62), for serving

sea salt (for garnish)

lime zest (for garnish)

orange zest (for garnish)

1. Slice lengthwise and remove the pits. (Don't cut the dates all the way through.)

2. Press the ends of each date toward each other to open the middle, and spoon in ½ teaspoon of almond butter.

3. Line the almond butter–filled dates on a serving platter and sprinkle with the spice blend.

4. Garnish with a few flakes of sea salt and zest right before serving.

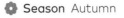 **Remedy tip** Dates stuffed in ghee make a deeply rejuvenative, nourishing treat. Instead of stuffing the date, you can stuff pitted dates in a glass jar three-quarters full of warmed Ghee (page 58). Set the jar aside to cool and enjoy a date a day for deep replenishment.

🌸 **Season** Autumn

🔻 **Dosha** Vata

Pistachio Truffles

30 MINUTES OR LESS

For these truffles, pistachios are blended into a melt-in-your-mouth cream, then rolled in a crunchy topping, creating sweet, creamy perfection for Autumn days when Vata winds begin to whip. You can get creative with the toppings. Alternate or mix the pistachio-orange-basil topping with raw cacao powder, shredded coconut, or a cinnamon-cardamom powder.

MAKES 6 TO 8 TRUFFLES

Prep time: 25 minutes

Cook time: 5 minutes

¾ cup raw unsalted pistachios, divided

1 tablespoon orange zest

3 or 4 basil leaves

1 tablespoon freshly squeezed orange juice, plus additional as needed

4 Medjool dates, pitted and roughly chopped

2 teaspoons coconut oil, divided, plus additional for rolling the dough

Pinch Autumn Spice Blend (page 62), plus additional as needed

Pinch salt (pink, mineral, or sea), plus additional as needed

1. Place ½ cup of pistachios in a small bowl and cover with water. Soak for 10 minutes. Drain the pistachios, rinse under cool water, and set on a towel to dry.

2. In a dry pan over medium heat, toast the remaining ¼ cup of pistachios for 5 minutes, stirring and tossing occasionally.

3. Transfer the toasted pistachios to a blender. Add the orange zest and basil, and pulse a few times to make a chunky blend. Transfer to a small bowl.

4. Put the soaked pistachios, orange juice, dates, 1 teaspoon of coconut oil, spice blend, and salt in the blender. Purée until smooth. Taste. If the mixture is too dry, blend in a little more orange juice or a drizzle of maple syrup. Adjust the seasonings, adding more spice blend or salt if necessary.

5. Lightly oil your hands with coconut oil. Roll a small handful of dough into a ball. Repeat until all the dough is rolled.

6. One at a time, roll the dough balls in the pistachio-orange-basil topping and place on a plate. Serve immediately, or refrigerate in an airtight container.

>>> **Preparation tip** To make it easier to roll the truffles, refrigerate the dough first for 15 minutes or up to 24 hours.

❀ **Season** Autumn

◐ **Dosha** Vata. For Pitta, replace pistachios with soaked almonds or pumpkin seeds.

Chocolate Pudding

30 MINUTES OR LESS

This pudding does not need to be cooked, baked, heated, or even chopped. It's a perfect dessert for Summer, or for those inevitable times when chocolate is the only answer. Food to console is food for your soul, and everyone knows a strong soul is essential to make a body whole. Garnish this pudding with blueberries and fresh mint. Or just dive in.

SERVES 2

Prep time: 5 minutes

1 avocado

2 tablespoons cacao powder

1 teaspoon vanilla extract

Large pinch ground cardamom

Drizzle maple syrup

Salt (pink, mineral, or sea), for seasoning

1. Scoop out the avocado and put it in a small electric blender.

2. Add the cacao powder, vanilla, cardamom, maple syrup, and salt, and mix until the pudding reaches a smooth consistency.

3. Taste and adjust the salt, cardamom, and syrup as needed.

⋙ **Remedy tip** This is a great vehicle for medicinal herbs or spices. If you feel you need turmeric, add a pinch. Cinnamon, add two pinches. I sometimes "hide" herbs like brahmi or tulsi in desserts loaded with good fats, much the way vets teach us to give our dogs medicine with peanut butter! The sweet taste helps the medicine go down.

✿ **Season** Summer. In Autumn, add a little additional cardamom and lightly warm the dessert by nestling the pudding bowl in a larger bowl of hot water for a few minutes before serving.

◐ **Dosha** Vata, Pitta. Not ideal for Kapha, but if so, choose honey to sweeten and cinnamon and cloves to warmly spice.

Nutty-Crusted Apple Pie

Nothing says Autumn like apple pie. As the pie bakes, the wafting aromas of caramelizing apples, cinnamon, and roasting pecans are the essence of warmth, whispering that all is okay in the world. Apples give a cooling energy, so this is balancing for Pitta, but good too for Vata and Kapha thanks to the nutty crust and warming spices. I recommend crisp apples such as Fuji, Gala, or Pink Lady for a contrasting taste of sweet and tart.

MAKES 8-10 SERVINGS

Prep time: 20 minutes
Cook time: 30 minutes

FOR THE PIECRUST

2 cups pecans

10 Medjool dates, pitted

1 tablespoon Ghee (page 58)

Large pinch
ground cinnamon

Pinch ground nutmeg

Pinch salt
(pink, mineral, or sea)

FOR THE PIE FILLING

2 tablespoons lemon juice

1 tablespoon maple syrup

1 teaspoon vanilla extract

1 teaspoon Ghee, melted

½ teaspoon Autumn Spice Blend (page 62)

5 apples, cored and sliced

Raw honey (for serving)

TO MAKE THE PIECRUST

1. Preheat the oven to 350°F.

2. Toast the pecans in a sauté pan over medium-high heat until they begin to brown. Stir in the ghee.

3. Put the dates, cinnamon, nutmeg, and salt in a blender and pulse to combine.

4. Add the pecans to the blender and pulse enough to break up the pecans, and be careful not to make pecan butter.

5. Transfer the mixture to a 9-inch pie pan and press the crust evenly across the bottom and up along the sides of the pan.

6. Bake for 5 minutes. Set aside to cool.

TO MAKE THE PIE FILLING

1. Whisk the lemon juice, maple syrup, vanilla extract, ghee, and spices together in a large bowl.

2. Add the apple slices to the bowl and toss gently.

3. Starting with one apple slice at the center of the piecrust, arrange the slices in a tight spiral to create a rose petal pattern. Layer the apple slices until the entire pie is covered, and then sprinkle the remaining juice from the bowl over the top.

4. Cover the pie with foil and bake for about 30 minutes, or until the apples are soft. Let cool for 5 minutes, and then flip the pie onto a serving plate.

5. Drizzle the pie with raw honey. If you wish, you can also garnish the pie with rosemary, mint, or pomegranate seeds. Serve, optionally, with a thick yogurt.

≫ **Cooking tip** For a sweeter pie, sprinkle handfuls of raisins, dried cherries, or chocolate chips evenly over the crust and then layer the apple slices on top before baking.

✿ **Season** Autumn, Winter

◬ **Dosha** Vata. Pitta. Okay in moderation for Kapha.

Carrot Halva

ONE POT

Halva can be made from beets, pumpkins, or any sweet and starchy fruit or root, making it a great way to serve up vital plant nutrients to veggie dodgers. Make it with your favorite milk—almond, rice, or coconut—but make sure you cook long enough to boil off the water and get a thick pudding. This halva is delicious with honey yogurt for a midday dessert, or even with ginger tea for a light, sweet supper.

SERVES 4

Prep time: 5 minutes

Cook time: 1 hour

1 tablespoon Ghee (page 58)

1 teaspoon Autumn Spice Blend (page 62) or Winter Spice Blend (page 63)

½ cup cashews

4 large carrots, grated

½ cup raisins

1 cup whole milk

¼ cup water

Maple syrup, jaggery, or coconut sugar, if needed

1. Melt the ghee in a saucepan over medium heat. Stir in the spice blend and swirl the pan to combine. Add the cashews and cook for 3 minutes, stirring occasionally.

2. Stir in the carrots, raisins, milk, and water to the pan and bring to a boil. Reduce the heat to low, cover the pan, and simmer for 1 hour, or until the liquid is absorbed.

3. Taste. Stir in maple syrup, if needed, and serve warm.

⤳ **Substitution tip** For a Pitta-balancing treat, peel and grate beets instead of carrots, and replace the cashews with sliced almonds.

❀ **Season** Autumn, Winter

◈ **Dosha** Vata

Coconut-Mango Crumble

Light and caramelly, this crumble is a pure taste of Summer. Be sure to use ripe mangos for a juicy, syrupy filling that delightfully balances the light crunch of the topping. While the recipe calls for ½ cup of sugar, it measures out to only about 1 tablespoon per serving, making it healthy enough to enjoy this dessert for breakfast.

SERVES 8

Prep time: 15 minutes

Cook time: 30 minutes

¼ cup Homemade Coconut Milk (page 66)

2 tablespoons freshly squeezed lime juice

4 cups chopped mangos (3 to 4 mangos)

3 tablespoons maple syrup, divided

2 teaspoons vanilla extract

Salt (pink, mineral, or sea), for seasoning

½ cup shredded coconut

½ cup coconut sugar

1 teaspoon ground cardamom

¼ cup coconut oil

1. In a small bowl, combine the coconut milk with 1 tablespoon of lime juice, and set aside to sour.

2. Preheat the oven to 350°F.

3. In a large bowl, mix the mangos, 1 tablespoon of maple syrup, the vanilla, the remaining lime juice, and a pinch of salt.

4. Pour the filling into a standard pie dish or an 8-by-8-inch baking dish, and spread evenly.

5. In a medium bowl, stir together the shredded coconut, coconut sugar, cardamom, and a few pinches of salt. Work the coconut oil in with your hands until the mixture is completely moistened, then lightly stir in the remaining 2 tablespoons of maple syrup and the soured coconut milk.

6. Crumble this coconut mixture over the mango filling and bake for 30 minutes, or until the fruit bubbles and the topping lightly browns.

>>> **Serving tip** Serve for breakfast with fresh berries or bananas, or enjoy as an afternoon snack with a dollop of yogurt and fresh mint. Drizzle with honey if you like extra sweetness.

✿ **Seasons** Summer, early Autumn

◈ **Doshas** Vata, Pitta

Healthy Hot Chocolate

ONE POT • 30 MINUTES OR LESS

This guilt-free hot chocolate recipe comes from my friend, the herbalist health educator, and co-founder of the San Diego Herb Company, Nicole Plaisted, who says, "Cacao nourishes our brain, heart, nerves, and bones to keep us looking young and feeling great while subtly helping stave off disease." Ironically, Ayurveda cautions us that chocolate, with its pungent and bitter tastes, can aggravate Vata and Pitta. The addition of coconut milk and maple syrup mitigates those tastes and gives a balancing sweetness for holidays and quiet nights by the fire that call for a special treat. The truth is, chocolate can transport us from peeved to passionate in one time-stopping, evocative bite—and that itself is good medicine.

MAKES 2 CUPS

Prep time: 5 minutes

Cook time: 10 minutes

2 cups Homemade Coconut Milk (page 66)

3 to 4 tablespoons cacao powder

1 teaspoon maple syrup, plus more as needed

3 or 4 pinches ground cinnamon

2 shakes grated nutmeg

Bring the coconut milk to a boil in a small saucepan. Stir in the cacao powder, maple syrup, cinnamon, and nutmeg. If it is too thick for your taste, add water to reach your desired consistency. Pour into mugs and enjoy.

⇾⇾ **Remedy tip** Ayurveda believes medicinal components are made more bioavailable when combined with a healthy fat and delivered with the sweet taste, making this a great vehicle for medicinal herbs and spices. Add a teaspoon of turmeric, ginger, triphala, ashwagandha, or any powdered herbs you are currently prescribed, as the coconut milk is boiling.

✿ **Season** Autumn, Winter. In Summer, replace the cinnamon with 2 pinches of ground cardamom.

◭ **Dosha** Vata, Pitta, with the Summer replacement mentioned previously.

Easy Homemade Jam

30 MINUTES OR LESS

Psyllium is a powerful binder, which is one reason it is so popular as a dietary fiber supplement. Psyllium fiber comes from psyllium husk, and the names are used interchangeably. Look for it at your local grocer, usually found near the grains or in the supplements aisle. In this recipe, the psyllium acts like a gelatin, creating jam as fresh and easy as an early Summer morning. Spread on toast, spoon into breakfast bowls, stir into smoothies, or use it to dress up desserts.

MAKES 1 CUP

Prep time: 5 minutes

1 cup fresh Summer berries

1 tablespoon psyllium husks

1 tablespoon freshly squeezed lemon juice

Pinch salt (pink, mineral, or sea)

Place the berries, psyllium husks, lemon juice, and salt in a blender and pulse just enough for a chunky consistency.

Storage tip The jam will keep in an airtight container in the refrigerator up to 1 week, but it is best enjoyed at room temperature.

Season Year-round

Dosha Pitta. For Vata, stir into Nutty Oatmeal (page 85) or a warm bowl of grains. For Kapha, use to sweeten lighter grains like quinoa or amaranth.

Carrot Pickle, *page 185*, Lemony Ginger Chutney, *page 178*, Basil Pesto, *page 175*

eleven
Condiments, Spreads & Sauces

Cilantro Pesto 174

Basil Pesto 175

Apple Chutney 176

Coconut-Mint Chutney 177

Lemony Ginger Chutney 178

Preserved Lemons 179

Cucumber Raita 180

Pumpkin Seed Butter 181

Yogurt-Dill Dipping Sauce 182

Rice & Bean Hummus 183

Avocado Mash 184

Carrot Pickle 185

Cinnamon-Honey Syrup 186

Cilantro Pesto

30 MINUTES OR LESS • KITCHEN REMEDY

Cilantro is a popular herb used in cooking from Mexico to Thailand and regions all across India. Valued for its cooling properties, it has also been shown to help tissues chelate toxic metals. While Ayurveda usually avoids garlic, in this case the garlic aids in purification and boosts the flavor. Spoon this pesto over any savory dish for tasty healing benefits.

MAKES ¼ CUP

Prep time: 5 minutes

1 bunch cilantro

1 large garlic clove

2 tablespoons roasted pumpkin seeds

Juice of 1 lemon

Salt (pink, mineral, or sea), for seasoning

Freshly ground black pepper, for seasoning

Extra-virgin olive oil

1. Rinse the cilantro and pat dry. Pluck the leaves and put them in a blender with the garlic and pumpkin seeds. Pulse until chunky.

2. Add the lemon juice to the cilantro mixture. Pulse again until the pesto reaches your desired consistency.

3. Taste and adjust: If the pesto is too dry, add more lemon juice. If it is too runny, blend in more pumpkin seeds. Taste again and season with salt and pepper.

4. Spoon the pesto into a bowl and stir in a drizzle of olive oil.

>>> **Serving tip** Toss this pesto with pasta, stir it into soups and sautés, use it to add flavor to rice or kitchari, or enjoy it as a dip with crackers or sliced vegetables.

✿ **Season** Spring, Summer. In Autumn and Winter, add a handful of basil to the blender.

◭ **Dosha** Pitta, Kapha

Basil Pesto

30 MINUTES OR LESS · KITCHEN REMEDY

Basil Pesto is a versatile gem, beneficial for all doshas. It enhances flavor in every dish—great with pasta, "cheesy" when layered on top of baked dishes, and better than tomato sauce for a Flatbread Pizza (page 151). It can be served on toast, stirred into Avocado Mash (page 184), or spooned into any bowl of kitchari or soup for richer taste and digestive support.

MAKES 1 CUP

Prep time: 5 minutes

1 cup fresh basil leaves

1 tablespoon pine nuts

1 garlic clove

2 tablespoons extra-virgin olive oil

Pulse the basil, pine nuts, and garlic in a blender. Scrape the sides of the blender, and pulse again until you achieve a fine chop. Transfer to a small bowl and stir in the olive oil.

⋙ **Substitution tip** For a lighter, less expensive pesto, replace pine nuts with pumpkin seeds. For a cleansing pesto in Spring, add a handful of fresh parsley. Omit the garlic for Pitta.

✿ **Season** Spring, Summer

❀ **Dosha** All

Apple Chutney

Chutney is a condiment that makes it easy and quick to dress up rice, dals, stews, and sautés. With a crunchy play of sweet, sour, salty, astringent, and pungent, one spoonful of this chutney brings five of the six tastes to balance any meal. This recipe contrasts the cooling tart of apple with the spicy heat of the chili powder.

MAKES ½ CUP

Prep time: 3 minutes

1 crisp apple, cored and diced

1 tablespoon jaggery

½ teaspoon chili powder

1 teaspoon salt (pink, mineral, or sea)

1 to 2 tablespoons Hot & Spicy Oil (page 64)

1 teaspoon freshly squeezed lemon juice

Cilantro leaves, for garnish

Mix together the apple, jaggery, chili powder, salt, and oil in a small bowl. Stir in the lemon juice. Garnish with the cilantro.

Ingredient tip Made from dried cane juice, jaggery is considered a good medium for delivering Vata-balancing botanicals. It is richer but less sweet than sugar; in a pinch it can be replaced with coconut sugar.

Season Year-round

Dosha Kapha. Vata, Pitta in very small amounts.

Coconut-Mint Chutney

30 MINUTES OR LESS

In India, where it is mixed with pungent chiles, mint chutney is typically served with pakoras. This subtler version uses the heating energy of ginger to balance the cooling energy of mint. Coconut serves as a sweet base to the light, pungent spices. Stimulating to digestion, this chutney is excellent with heavier foods, and perfect with kitchari, any rice dishes, as a dip, and even as a salad dressing, thinned with extra-virgin olive oil.

MAKES ½ CUP

Prep time: 5 minutes
Cook time: 3 minutes

½ cup shredded coconut

1 (1½-inch) piece
fresh ginger

1 tablespoon warm water

¼ teaspoon salt

2 big handfuls fresh
mint leaves

1 tablespoon freshly
squeezed lime juice

1 teaspoon coconut oil

1 pinch brown mustard seeds

1. Mix the coconut, ginger, water, and salt in a blender.

2. Add the mint and lime juice and pulse to blend. Transfer to a small bowl.

3. Melt the coconut oil in a small saucepan over medium heat, and add the mustard seeds. As soon as the seeds begin to pop, remove the pan from heat. Stir the mustard seeds and oil into the coconut chutney.

>>> **Remedy tip** In cases of high heat, omit the ginger.

✿ **Season** Summer

🔱 **Dosha** Pitta, Vata

Lemony Ginger Chutney

Lemon is the bright sunshine that lifts and balances Vata. Ginger is the warmth that centers and grounds. Together, they make a dynamic duo of friendship for Vata, soothing digestion, easing nausea, hydrating tissue, and encouraging proper circulation. This sweet-sour chutney enlivens any dish and goes especially well with rice. With an extra drizzle of olive oil, it becomes a sunny marinade or a sweet salad dressing.

MAKES ½ CUP

Prep time: 5 minutes

2 tablespoons grated fresh ginger, plus any ginger juice from the grating process

¼ cup freshly squeezed lemon juice

1 tablespoon lemon zest

1 teaspoon jaggery, or coconut sugar

1 tablespoon extra-virgin olive oil

In a small bowl, stir together the ginger and ginger juice, lemon juice, lemon zest, jaggery, and olive oil. Store in an airtight jar in the refrigerator, but always serve at room temperature, or warm by sitting the jar in a bowl of hot water before serving.

Remedy tip Boost digestive fire by stirring 1 teaspoon of this chutney into dishes, or sip it with hot water as a tea.

Season Autumn

Dosha Vata

Preserved Lemons

KITCHEN REMEDY

Recently my sister helped me fulfill a longtime dream of having my own lemon tree, and now I get to enjoy the sunny gift of citrus all Winter long. Lemon's flowers and fragrance brighten any day, while its fruit brightens every dish. With a big citrusy, floral flavor, preserved lemons are the next best thing to having your own fresh lemons, available anytime, all year round, right in your own kitchen.

MAKES 2 CUPS

Prep time: 5 minutes, plus overnight to chill, and 1 month to preserve

4 to 5 lemons

¼ cup kosher salt

1. Slice the lemons crosswise into ½-inch-thick rounds. Place the slices in a large bowl and toss them with the salt.

2. Cover the bowl and refrigerate overnight.

3. The next day, stack the lemon slices inside a mason jar. Pour the liquid that accumulated in the bowl over the lemon slices and press the slices down to submerge them.

4. Seal the jar and store in a cool, dark place for 1 month or longer—preserved lemons get better with age. Shake every day, until the rinds are tender. Then refrigerate. Once preserved, the lemons will keep in the refrigerator for months.

5. To use, remove a piece of lemon and lightly rinse it. Serve with dishes as you would a slice of fresh lemon, or add it to kitchari, stews, or dal in the last 5 minutes of cooking.

>>> **Kitchen Remedy tip** Lightly fermented with notes of bitter from the peel, preserved lemon is a salty-sour dream for Vata, and a great way to bring sunny zest to Winter dishes. Add turmeric (root or powder), brown mustard seeds, cinnamon sticks, cloves, or black peppercorns to your jars before sealing to give your preserves even more of a medicinal charge.

❀ **Season** Autumn, Winter

◭ **Dosha** Vata. Use sparingly for Pitta, Kapha.

Cucumber Raita

Raita is standard in most Indian meals. You will usually find it next to the chutney and pickled carrots at Indian restaurants and homes. This trinity of peppery, pickled, and yogurt condiments improves the digestibility of meals. But one note: Yogurt is heavy and heating, and not advised for dinner, which should be light. Enjoy this raita with lunch, where it is creamy and refreshing on salads, in stews, with toast, and as a small side for savory mains.

MAKES 1½ CUPS

Prep time: 5 minutes

2 Persian cucumbers, peeled

1 medium carrot, shredded

1 cup plain yogurt

1 teaspoon ground ginger

1 handful cilantro, chopped

1. Quarter the cucumbers lengthwise, then slice them into quarter moons.

2. In a small bowl, combine the cucumbers, carrot, yogurt, ginger, and cilantro.

⋙ **Ingredient tip** Ayurveda tells us that the skin of fruit and vegetables helps nourish and heal our own skin. Rather than completely peeling the cucumbers, alternate the peel to leave stripes of green and white. The Persian cucumbers used here have a more delicate skin that you don't need to peel.

❀ **Season** Year-round

❋ **Dosha** All

Pumpkin Seed Butter

Pumpkin seed butter is a surprisingly nutty, satisfying alternative to peanut or almond butter. It can be stirred into soups or sautés for a rich sweet note, or spread onto slices of apple or banana for a healthy quick-energy snack. You can also add a spoonful to your smoothies or stir one into your breakfast oatmeal. With the Seasonal Fruit Compote (page 89), it's an Ayurvedic PBJ. Or eat it right off the spoon. It's that good.

MAKES 1 CUP

Prep time: 5 minutes, plus 6 hours to soak

1 cup pumpkin seeds

½ cup sunflower seeds

1 tablespoon raw honey

2 shakes ground cinnamon

Pinch ground ginger

Pinch pink salt

1. Put the pumpkin seeds and sunflower seeds in a small bowl. Cover with water by a couple of inches. Soak the seeds for 6 to 8 hours or overnight.

2. Drain the seeds and pat them dry on a towel.

3. Put the seeds in a blender along with the honey, cinnamon, ginger, and salt. Blend until creamy.

4. Store in an airtight jar in a dark place.

Remedy tip Ayurvedic lore says that for strong reproductive tissue and regenerative energy, you should eat seeds, as in pumpkin seeds, sunflower seeds, and flaxseed. Additionally, pumpkin seeds purify and nourish, making this a delicious rejuvenative remedy.

Season Year-round

Dosha Pumpkin seeds are lighter than peanuts or tree nuts. Their astringent quality supports cleansing and elimination/purification, making them good for Kapha, while their nutrition profile makes them nourishing for Vata and Pitta.

Yogurt-Dill Dipping Sauce

30 MINUTES OR LESS

This dip is wonderful with crackers or hot Chapatis (page 69), or with fresh vegetables and salads. Or, like most of the recipes in this chapter, it is great stirred into rice for a simple, nourishing meal. You can also add parsley, mint, or cilantro for a thicker, emerald-dappled dip. Or thin it with extra-virgin olive oil for a digestion-enhancing dressing.

MAKES 1½ CUPS

Prep time: 5 minutes

1 bunch dill

1 cup plain yogurt

1 teaspoon mayonnaise

Juice of 1 lime

Salt (pink, mineral, or sea), for seasoning

Freshly ground black pepper, for seasoning

1. Finely chop the dill and transfer it to a medium bowl.

2. Add the yogurt, mayonnaise, and lime juice, and whisk to combine. Season with salt and pepper.

⋙ **Substitution tip** Stir with a pinch celery salt and a drizzle of extra-virgin olive oil for a creamy salad dressing. Replace the yogurt with creamy Paneer (page 100) for a Summer veggie dip.

✿ **Season** Autumn. Summer when paired with raw vegetables or salads for lunch.

❋ **Dosha** Vata. For Pitta, use paneer instead of yogurt.

Rice & Bean Hummus

30 MINUTES OR LESS

Turn everyday hummus into a royal snack by blending your kitchari with lemon juice and tahini. It elevates the classic rice and beans to a creamy party dish, delicious with crisp vegetables in Summer and savory sautés in Autumn, Winter, and Spring.

MAKES 1 CUP

Prep time: 5 minutes

1 cup Seasonal Kitchari

1 tablespoon tahini

3 hearty shakes cayenne

1 tablespoon freshly squeezed lemon juice

1 tablespoon extra-virgin olive oil

Salt (pink, mineral, or sea), for seasoning

Freshly ground black pepper, for seasoning

1. Put the kitchari, tahini, cayenne, and lemon juice in a blender. Purée until you achieve your desired consistency, whether chunky or creamy.

2. Drizzle in the olive oil and pulse the blender quickly a few times to gently blend it with the hummus.

3. Season with salt and pepper. Serve as a dip with fresh vegetables.

↠ **Serving tip** Excellent stirred in with Creamy Quinoa (page 86). Or for Vata/Autumn, serve with Tahini Yogurt (page 113); for Pitta/Summer on a bed of romaine.

❋ **Season** Spring. For Summer, replace the cayenne with dried dill, mint, or basil.

◈ **Dosha** Kapha. For Pitta, use the Summer substitutes above.

Avocado Mash

30 MINUTES OR LESS

Make a simple but sumptuous dinner in minutes by lathering Avocado Mash over piping-hot Chapatis (page 69). Or spoon generous amounts of Avocado Mash onto your Kitchari "Burgers" (page 144) or into your Rice & Bean Burritos (page 148). Thin the mash with extra-virgin olive oil and another spoonful of lime juice, and it becomes a rich dressing for Summer salads. You can replace the mayonnaise with vegan mayonnaise or a silken tofu.

SERVES 2

Prep time: 5 minutes

1 avocado, pitted

1 tablespoon mayonnaise

1 tablespoon freshly squeezed lime juice

Salt (pink, mineral, or sea), for seasoning

Freshly ground black pepper, for seasoning

1. In a small bowl, mash the avocado. Stir in the mayonnaise and lime juice.

2. Season lightly with salt and pepper.

⋙ **Ingredient tip** Choose avocados that lightly give when pressed. Slice in half lengthwise to open. With a knife, stab the pit hard with the bottom of the blade and give it a twist to remove it. Scoop out the flesh with a spoon.

⬢ **Season** Summer

◭ **Dosha** Vata, Pitta

Carrot Pickle

KITCHEN REMEDY

Carrot Pickle is an easy-to-make, fast fermented food. All you need is a wide-mouth mason jar with a lid and band, some whey, water, salt, and a dark, warm (72°F) area, plus 2 or 3 days for the fermentation. Whey is the liquid that remains from making Paneer (page 100). It is a milk product, so if you're dairy-free, simply omit the whey and leave the carrots to ferment another day or two.

MAKES 2 CUPS CARROT PICKLE AND 4 CUPS BRINE

Prep time: 5 minutes, plus 2 days to ferment

2 tablespoons whey

2 tablespoons kosher salt

6 carrots, shredded

1 beet, peeled and grated, and its juices

1 (1-inch) piece fresh ginger, peeled and cut into rounds

1 teaspoon brown mustard seeds

Filtered water

1. Sterilize a large mason jar by pouring boiling water in and over it. Pour out the water.

2. Put the whey and salt in the jar, and stir briskly to dissolve the salt. Add the carrots, beet, ginger, and mustard seeds and stir again.

3. Fill the jar to the neck with the filtered water. Cover the jar with a clean dish towel, and set aside in a warm, dark place.

4. After 2 days, check the pickle. If the carrot tastes pickled, it is done. If not, re-cover and let stand for 1 more day. By day 3, it should be done. Serve, or seal with the lid and band and store in the refrigerator.

⋙ **Kitchen Remedy tip** The liquid (the brine) makes a probiotic drink you can sip or add to smoothies.

✿ **Season** Autumn, Winter

◭ **Dosha** Vata

Cinnamon-Honey Syrup

KITCHEN REMEDY

As the Ayurvedic sage Charak wrote thousands of years ago, "Let your kitchen be your first pharmacy," your pantry really is full of medicine. This homemade syrup is one of many examples. For a sore throat or dry throat, take ½ teaspoon of this syrup every hour. For coughs or heavy mucus, stir it into warm water with 1 tablespoon of lemon juice to make a tea, and sip throughout the day. To strengthen digestion, take a spoonful before meals.

MAKES ¼ CUP

Prep time: 10 minutes, plus 30 minutes to sit

4 tablespoons raw honey

1 fresh ginger knob, peeled and minced

½ teaspoon ground cinnamon

½ teaspoon ground cloves

1 tablespoon freshly squeezed lemon juice

1. Spoon the honey into a small bowl. Fill a larger bowl with hot water and nestle the smaller bowl in the larger bowl.

2. Once the honey softens, remove the small bowl from the water. Stir in the ginger, cinnamon, and cloves. Add the lemon juice and stir well. Let this sit for 30 minutes for the lemon to thin the honey.

3. Store in an airtight container at room temperature.

⫸ **Kitchen Remedy tip** For a weight-loss tonic, replace the cloves with freshly ground black pepper and double the amount of lemon juice, then stir 1 tablespoon of the syrup into a tall glass of warm water. Sip at 15-minute intervals during the day.

✿ **Season** Year-round, especially Winter, Spring

❀ **Dosha** Kapha

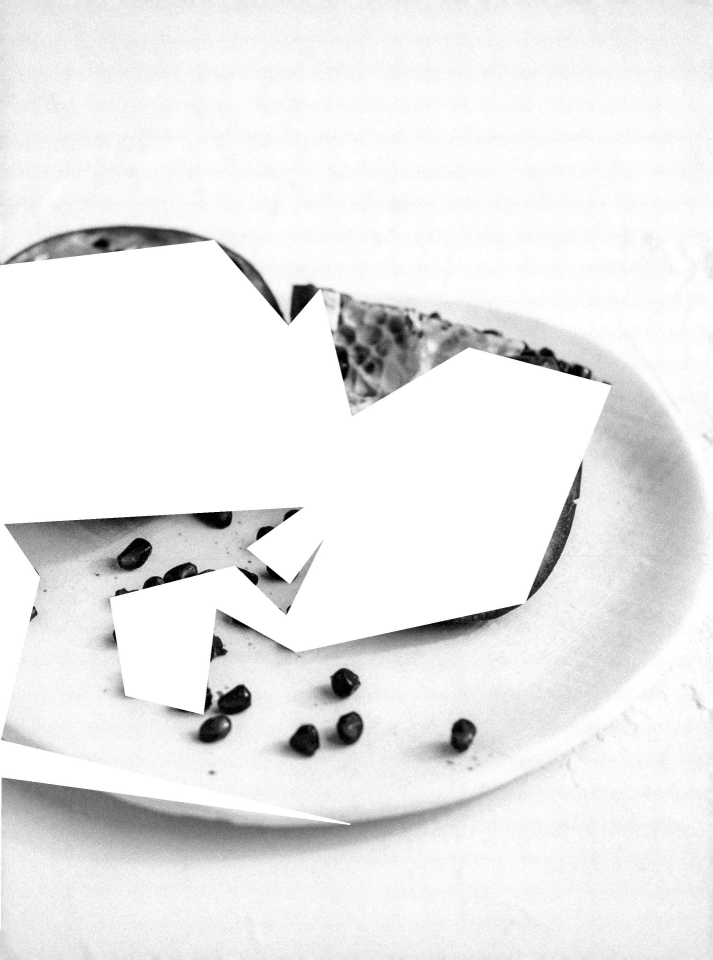

An In-Depth Look at Doshic States

While the five elements make up all of the natural world, existing and moving within and all around us, each of us is born with a unique combination of the elements that gives a tendency toward one constitutional dosha: Vata, Pitta, or Kapha. The key to balance, wellness, and healing is to monitor your dosha throughout your life, understanding, too, that doshas fluctuate. You can have a constitutional dosha, which is a lifelong tendency, and you can have a different, or current, doshic imbalance.

Doshic Balance: Quick Summary

- Vata needs fire and water, which are warming and grounding.
- Pitta needs air and water, which are flowing and cooling.
- Kapha needs air and fire, which are circulating and igniting.

This appendix has lists of foods, spices, and meal preparation guidelines to balance each dosha. In applying these guidelines, consider the current imbalance, and try not to disturb the constitutional dosha. For instance, a Vata imbalance will need to ground, lubricate, and warm. But a Pitta constitution with a Vata imbalance will need to not increase internal heat. The dual dosha list will help with that. Remember, too, that for everyday wellness the guidelines are simple: six tastes at every meal, with ingredients and preparation aligned with the season.

Vata

Vata is air with space, giving dynamism, lightness, quick thinking, and intuition. Positive Vata is full of energy, creativity, curiosity, and inspiration. Imbalanced Vata can be dry, rough, jittery, ungrounded, scattered, or spacey.

You are Vata if…

- You are tall, or small and thin, with prominent, stiff, or creaky joints.
- Your hair is curly, your skin is dry, and your feet are cold.
- You are energetic, highly creative, and curious about the world.
- You love to move, travel, and explore.
- You enjoy new experiences, excitement, and stimulation.
- You are flexible and adaptable to new situations.
- You love to meet people and learn new things.

DIETARY RECOMMENDATIONS FOR VATA DOSHA

When Vata is dominant, focus on the tastes sweet, sour, and salty, and include foods that are liquid or unctuous like healthy fats, soups, and nut milks to balance dryness; "heavy" foods like root vegetables or bananas to offer sustained nourishment; foods that are smooth, like avocados, to offset roughness; and foods that are warm like ginger and radishes to balance the cool nature of Vata.

Cooked: Meals should be hot or warm. Puréed soups, cooked fruit, hot cereal, rice pudding, and hot beverages such as nut milks or warm milk are excellent comfort foods. Avoid or minimize raw foods such as salads and raw sprouts. Raw food is light, dry, rough, and hard to digest, so it aggravates Vata.

Grains: Rice, wheat, quinoa, oats, amaranth. Basmati rice is ideal, especially cooked with a little salt and ghee, or even milk. Whole-wheat flour, for chapatis, drizzled with melted ghee, is strengthening and balances well with cooked vegetables or a mild chutney.

Vegetables: Carrots, asparagus, tender leafy greens, beets, sweet potatoes, parsnips, daikon, fresh peas, green beans, and Summer squash such as zucchini and yellow squash are good, and best when cooked with Vata-pacifying spices and served with grains or mung beans for a balanced meal. Avoid nightshades and larger beans.

Fruits: Avocados, pineapples, papayas, peaches, plums, grapes, mangos, oranges, cherries, all berries, limes and lemons, apples if stewed, coconut, fresh figs, and raisins (soaked).

Healthy Fats: Cook foods with a little ghee, which can be heated to high temperatures without affecting its nourishing, healing qualities. Use ghee to sauté vegetables or cook grains. Drizzle extra-virgin olive oil over fresh soft flatbreads, cooked grains, steamed greens. Avoid too many dry foods such as crackers, dry cold cereal, toast. Also avoid foods labeled "nonfat."

Nuts and Seeds: Heavy, oily, and unctuous, nuts are great for Vata, especially with spices. Almonds, walnuts, pecans, pistachios, hazelnuts, and cashews make good snacks tossed with cinnamon, curry, paprika, or a little salt. Sesame seeds are tonifying for Vata, as are sunflower, pumpkin, and poppy seeds. Soaked nuts and seeds can be blanched or roasted for warmth and toasty flavor. Nut milks with warming spices are excellent for Vata.

Dairy: Whole milk, cream, butter, fresh yogurt (stirred into foods and not taken cold), lassi, cottage cheese, fresh paneer.

Spices: Most spices are warming and enhance digestion. Especially balancing to Vata are fresh ginger, coriander, cardamom, nutmeg, cumin, cinnamon, basil, mustard seed, fennel, and fenugreek, with turmeric, ground ginger, and black pepper in smaller quantities.

Vata people love to be free, so let yourself be creative, but be sure to create consistency, regularity, and stability as much as you can. You will feel the difference. Seek warm, nourishing people and experiences, just as you do with your food. Ghee is lubricating and rejuvenating. Add ghee to honey for a daily moisturizer or mix it with avocado for a rejuvenating mask. A full-body massage with sesame oil every morning before showering is instrumental for Vata.

Rest after work with your legs up the wall, hips elevated on a towel or blanket, and take deep, long, slow breaths. Drink warm almond milk with nutmeg at night to help with sleep, and no digital devices after dinner. Soak in an Epsom salts bath with lavender essential oil before bed.

Quick summary: To keep Vata in balance, consistently cultivate slow, warm, grounding, nourishing qualities in your meals, your friends, your activities, your breath, your mind, your life.

Pitta

Pitta is fire with some water, giving clarity, radiance, vision, and passion. Positive Pitta is warm, courageous, focused, insightful, and discerning. Imbalanced Pitta can be hot, oily, inflamed, intense, irritated, and impatient.

You are Pitta if…

- You are strong, with reddish, warm skin.
- Your eyes are piercing, and you have fine or straight hair.
- You have good circulation and are usually warm.
- You have a good appetite, sharp memory, and speech.
- You are motivated, warm, determined, and brave.
- You have a strong will, enjoy challenges, and face obstacles head-on.

DIETARY RECOMMENDATIONS FOR PITTA DOSHA

When Pitta is dominant, focus on the sweet, bitter, and astringent tastes. Include sweet foods to soothe Pitta, like stone fruits, roasted root vegetables, coconut; dry foods like beans, apples, cauliflower, green tea, and turmeric to balance the liquid nature of Pitta; dense and grounding foods like grains, root vegetables, milk, seeds, and cooling oils that offer sustained nourishment; and cooling foods like cucumbers, melons, and mint to balance the fiery quality of Pitta.

Cooling: Apples, pears, peaches, pomegranates, and sweet juicy fruits cool a fiery Pitta. Summer vegetables, dairy and nut milks, rice pudding, coconut, and smoothies made with mangos, almonds, or dates are examples of Pitta-cooling foods.

Grains: Basmati rice, wheat, barley, oats, amaranth, all cooked until tender, are balancing for Pitta. Whole-wheat flour, for chapatis or breakfast porridge, is a good dense food for Pitta. Dry cereal, crackers, granola, and rice cakes balance the liquid nature of Pitta.

Lentils: Whole and split mung beans, red and brown lentils, small portions of chickpeas, lima beans, black beans, pinto beans.

Vegetables: Asparagus, tender lettuces, bitter leafy greens, bitter gourd, carrots, celery, green beans, peas, zucchini, squash, cucumber, artichoke, okra, fennel, Brussels sprouts, broccoli, cauliflower, beets, sweet potatoes, parsnips—sweetened by cooking, grilling, sautéing, or roasting—are excellent with rice and dal for sustenance and balance. Avoid nightshades.

Fruits: Avocados, pineapples, peaches, plums, grapes, mangos, melons, pears, pomegranates, cherries, all berries, apples, coconut, dates, fresh and dried figs, and soaked raisins make good snacks for Pitta, the only dosha who may need something between meals for hunger pains.

Healthy Oils: Ghee is cooling for body and mind. It is the best oil for cooking, as it can be heated to high temperatures without affecting its nourishing, healing qualities. Use ghee to sauté vegetables, cook grains, slather on breads, and stir into warm drinks. Use extra-virgin olive oil for cool-temperature meals.

Nuts and Seeds: Nuts are oily for Pitta and generally discouraged with the exception of almonds, soaked and blanched. Sunflower seeds and pumpkin seeds are good alternatives to nuts and add a healthy crunch to salads, soups, and dal.

Dairy: Whole milk, cream, ghee, lassi, cottage cheese, and fresh paneer are cooling and soothing for Pitta.

Spices: Pitta-balancing spices enhance digestion without heating. Mint, fennel, dill, and small quantities of turmeric, cumin, coriander, cinnamon, cardamom, and basil offer flavor, aroma, and healing wisdom. Turmeric, coriander, small quantities of black pepper, Chinese cinnamon, saffron, sweet orange zest, cilantro, curry leaves, parsley, fresh basil, fresh fennel, and fresh mint.

LIFESTYLE

While Pitta loves vigorous, challenging exercise, walking, hiking, biking, swimming, and slow Yoga are best. Space and air balance Pitta, so seek expansive vistas and flowing movements.

Breathe deep when things get intense, and focus on long, smooth exhales. Water is cooling, so splash your face or soak your feet in cold water when feeling hot and bothered.

Eyes relate to the liver, which is the prime organ of Pitta in the body, so start your day with a good eye wash to cool and soothe internal Pitta. Cup your hand, fill it with room-temperature purified water, and bring it to your eye. Keep your eye open and let it bathe in the water until the water drips away. Repeat five times for each eye.

Fire gives light and light creates color, making Pitta people great visionaries and colorful storytellers. Surround yourself with the colors green, blue, and white. Green is the color of forests, nature, and prana, so it is healing for Pitta. Blue, the color of water and open skies, is cooling. White, the color of snow, is purifying and spacious. Visualizing these colors in your meditation or as you fall asleep is calming for the Pitta mind.

Quick summary: To keep Pitta in balance, cultivate cool, sweet, soothing balance in your meals and activities.

Kapha

Kapha is water with some earth, giving strength, stability, reliability, and calm. Positive Kapha is nurturing, forgiving, patient, generous, and grounding. Imbalanced Kapha is stagnant, muddy, stuck, stubborn, heavy, possessive, and melancholic.

You are Kapha if…

- You are grounded, strong, and stable.

- You have thick wavy hair, strong nails, and milky skin.

- You are considered calm, steady, and nurturing.

- You prefer a cozy home and familiar routines.

- You like traditions, are happy with a few close friends, and avoid risks.

- You are loyal, loving, and caring, and have a great memory.

DIETARY RECOMMENDATIONS FOR KAPHA DOSHA

When Kapha is dominant, focus on the pungent, bitter, and astringent tastes. Choose foods that are nourishing but light, like dark leafy greens, berries, and seeds, to counter the heaviness of Kapha. Include a few dry foods (like beans, toast, and persimmons) in your daily diet to balance the oily nature of Kapha and focus on warm, pungent foods (like ginger and peppers) and Spring greens (like watercress and arugula) to balance the sweet, cold quality of Kapha.

Avoid Sugar: Have an apple if you crave sweet, or spicy popcorn if you crave a treat. Use raw honey in moderation, and never heated, as your sweetener.

Light and Warm: Clear vegetable soups with beans and diced vegetables, steamed vegetables or stews, bean casseroles, mung dal, and light grain and vegetable combinations are ideal, especially when combined with Kapha-balancing spices. Reduce salt and avoid oily foods.

Grains: Choose lighter whole grains and eat them in moderation. Barley, buckwheat, quinoa, millet, oats, amaranth, sago, small portions of basmati rice, all cooked until tender. Dry cereal, salt-free crackers, rice cakes, and toast balance the liquid nature of Kapha.

Lentils: Mung beans, dal, red or brown lentils, small portions of chickpeas, lima beans, black beans, all cooked until butter-soft.

Vegetables: Asparagus, all leafy greens, bitter gourd, green beans, squash, artichokes, celery, Brussels sprouts, broccoli, cauliflower, beets, kohlrabi, daikon, radishes, and cabbage should be cooked with Kapha-pacifying spices.

Fruits: Apricots, prunes, peaches, pears, cherries, berries, apples, lemons, limes, pomegranates, dried figs, and raisins have astringent qualities to balance the sweet for Kapha.

Healthy Oils: Reduce oils and oily foods. In very small quantities, ghee is your best cooking oil.

Nuts and Seeds: Avoid nuts. Choose sunflower, pumpkin, sesame seeds instead.

Dairy: Dilute whole milk with water. Add spices to lassi, small portions of cottage cheese, or fresh paneer.

Spices: Pungent spices are wonderful for balancing Kapha, Ginger, cinnamon, cloves, cumin, coriander, cayenne, red pepper flakes, black pepper, green chiles, mustard seeds, fenugreek, turmeric, and fresh herbs like parsley, basil, mint, oregano, thyme, rosemary, and sage enhance flavor while improving digestion and circulation.

LIFESTYLE

For optimal health, give yourself a digestion rest one day a week by preparing stewed apples with ginger and cinnamon for breakfast, kitchari for lunch, and steamed vegetables or vegetable soup for dinner.

Air and fire balance Kapha, so move, circulate, meet new people, try new things, volunteer at a local service organization, or sign up for a new course.

Kapalabhati is a great Pranayama practice for Kapha. You could do 36 rounds each morning before you meditate to energize body and mind. Google it to learn how.

Visualizing red and orange in your meditation or as you fall asleep are balancing for your mind.

Quick summary: To keep Kapha in balance, cultivate light, warm, and stimulating qualities in your meals, and in everyday life.

Dual Doshas

At the level of healing a serious illness, a skilled Ayurvedic doctor will determine an underlying dosha as a cause to be treated. It can be tricky, because sometimes symptoms look like one dosha, but the actual problem is with another. As an example, fire consumes air. So a Pitta imbalance can look like a Vata expression. A person who has had too much sun can have dry, rough skin. A person who has "fried their brain" can have cognitive impairment. A person who is "burned out" may feel scattered or depleted. Or, Pitta inflammation can cause swelling, stagnation, or digestive dysfunction that can look like a Kapha disorder.

Those of us who are still refining our skills of subtle perception might experience that as a dual dosha. If you have a serious condition, please consult an experienced Ayurvedic doctor. The following guidelines are for general everyday wellness.

VATA-PITTA

If Vata and Pitta are dominant in your constitution, you express the elements of space, air, and fire. While the qualities of Vata are dry, light, cool, rough, subtle, and mobile, the qualities of Pitta are oily, sharp, hot, light, fleshy smelling, spreading, and liquid. The common qualities are light and subtle, so Vata-Pitta needs earth and water for grounding and nurturing.

Choose foods with the qualities of heavy like cheese, dense like sweet potatoes, slow like paneer, stable like wheat, and soft like rice. Bananas, roasted root vegetables, dal, rice pudding, chapatis, Summer fruit smoothies with cardamom and almond milk, and ghee are examples of Vata-Pitta-balancing foods.

In fact, the staple Ayurvedic diet of kitchari, basmati rice, mung dal, steamed vegetables with ghee, and lightly cooked fruit, is ideal for Vata-Pitta types.

Follow Vata guidelines at the change of seasons, in Autumn and Winter, and when the weather turns cold. Follow Pitta guidelines during the late Spring and Summer and whenever the weather is warm and moist.

VATA-KAPHA

If Vata and Kapha are dominant in your constitution, you express the elements of space, air, water, and earth. While the qualities of Vata are dry, light, cool, rough, subtle, and mobile, the qualities of Kapha are unctuous, cool, heavy, slow, smooth, soft, stable, dense, and cloudy.

What is missing is fire. Vata and Kapha are both cold, so they need warmth. Foods support their reduced digestive fire and *agni*-enhancing spices.

Choose foods with the qualities of hot, like ginger, daikon, mustard greens, and watercress. Cook all your foods, generously spice, and serve warm. Follow the guidelines for daily meals eating light and cooked in the morning, eating your main meal at lunchtime, and eating light and soupy for dinner. Ginger-lemon tea with meals will enhance digestion, and the occasional lassi will help move things along.

The staple Ayurvedic diet of kitchari, steamed vegetables, and clear soups is good for Vata-Kapha types. Follow Vata guidelines at the change of seasons, in Autumn and Winter, and when the weather is windy and dry. Follow Kapha guidelines during the Spring and anytime the weather is heavy and wet.

PITTA-KAPHA

If Pitta and Kapha are dominant in your constitution, you express the elements of fire, water, and earth. While the qualities of Pitta are oily, sharp, hot, light, fleshy smelling, spreading, and liquid, the qualities of Kapha are unctuous, cool, heavy, slow, smooth, soft, stable, dense, and cloudy.

The common element is water, so Pitta-Kapha needs air and space to lift and elevate, circulate, and flow. Choose foods that are drying, like legumes, celery, sweet potatoes, apples, pomegranates, quinoa, barley, dry crackers, and toast.

The Ayurvedic staples of kitchari, mung dal, and steamed leafy greens and vegetables, with reduced amounts of ghee, are ideal for Pitta-Kapha types.

Follow Pitta guidelines during the Summer and whenever the weather is warm. Follow Kapha guidelines during late Winter and Spring, and whenever the weather is cold.

Tri-doshic

Vata-Pitta-Kapha types have the three doshas evenly in their constitutions. It is rare, but it means the doshas nearly balance each other out. In this case, your very best guidance is to follow the seasons. In Spring, eat light, cooked, and pungent. In Summer, eat fresh, cooling foods with mint and dill. In Autumn, grounding grains, dals, and roasted root vegetables are balancing. And in Winter, warm spicy soups are best.

Tri-doshic people will be warm, creative, and grounded. If you find yourself feeling out of balance, look to the imbalanced dosha and apply the guidelines lightly so one dosha doesn't cause an imbalance in another.

Once you understand the elements and how they play out through the doshas, you gain an intuitive understanding of your needs. From there, you get to enjoy sacred, sumptuous living with ease.

Seasonal & Dosha-Balancing Food Lists

In seed time learn, in harvest teach, in Winter enjoy.

—WILLIAM BLAKE

Stock your pantry from the following All Seasons list, and consult the seasonal lists for fresh, dosha-balancing ingredients.

All Seasons

FRUITS

- Coconut, shredded
- Lemons, limes
- Raisins

VEGETABLES

- Carrots
- Celery
- Green beans
- Leafy greens
- Sweet potatoes
- Zucchini

GRAINS

- Basmati rice
- Oats
- Quinoa

LEGUMES

- Fava beans
- Whole mung beans, split

NUTS AND SEEDS

- Almonds
- Cashews
- Chia seeds
- Flaxseed
- Pumpkin seeds
- Sesame seeds

OILS

- Coconut oil
- Extra-virgin olive oil
- Ghee

HERBS

- Basil
- Cilantro
- Parsley

SPICES

- Black pepper
- Cardamom, ground
- Cinnamon, ground
- Coriander seed
- Fennel seed
- Fenugreek, ground
- Ginger, fresh
- Nutmeg, whole
- Salt, pink
- Salt, sea
- Tamari
- Turmeric

SWEETENERS

- Honey
- Jaggery
- Maple syrup

Spring Shopping List

FRUITS

- Apples
- Apricots
- Blueberries
- Cherries
- Cranberries
- Currants
- Dried fruit
- Lemons
- Limes
- Peaches
- Pears
- Pomegranates
- Prunes
- Raisins
- Raspberries

VEGETABLES

- Artichoke
- Arugula
- Asparagus
- Beets and beet greens
- Broccoli
- Brussels sprouts
- Cabbage
- Carrots
- Cauliflower
- Celery
- Chard
- Chicory
- Chiles
- Collard greens
- Daikon
- Dandelion greens
- Endive
- Escarole
- Green beans
- Lettuce
- Mustard greens
- Nettles
- Peas
- Radicchio
- Radishes
- Spinach
- Sprouts
- Sweet potatoes
- Turnips
- Watercress

GRAINS

- Amaranth
- Barley
- Basmati rice
- Buckwheat
- Corn
- Millet
- Oats (dry)
- Quinoa
- Rice cakes
- Rye
- Seitan
- Tapioca

LEGUMES

- Adzuki beans
- Bean sprouts
- Black beans
- Black-eyed peas
- Chickpeas
- Kidney beans
- Lentils
- Lima beans
- Miso
- Mung beans, split
- Mung beans, whole
- Navy beans
- Pinto beans
- Tempeh
- White beans

SEEDS

- Pumpkin seeds
- Sesame seeds
- Sunflower seeds

DAIRY

- Cottage cheese
- Feta
- Yogurt

OILS

- Extra-virgin olive oil
- Ghee
- Mustard oil

SWEETENERS

- Honey, raw
- Molasses

SPICES

- Basil
- Black pepper
- Cayenne
- Chiles
- Cinnamon
- Ginger
- Oregano
- Parsley
- Red pepper flakes
- Tarragon
- Thyme
- Turmeric

Summary Shopping List

FRUITS

- Apples
- Avocados
- Blackberries
- Blueberries
- Cherries
- Coconut
- Cranberries
- Grapes
- Limes
- Mangos
- Melons
- Nectarines
- Peaches
- Pears
- Pineapples
- Plums
- Pomegranates
- Prunes
- Raspberries
- Strawberries
- Watermelons

VEGETABLES

- Artichokes
- Arugula
- Asparagus
- Beet greens
- Bok choy
- Broccoli
- Brussels sprouts
- Cabbage
- Cauliflower
- Celery
- Chard
- Collard greens
- Cucumbers
- Green beans
- Kale
- Lettuce
- Summer squash
- Sweet potatoes
- Zucchini

GRAINS

- Amaranth
- Barley
- Basmati rice
- Couscous
- Quinoa
- Wheat

LEGUMES

- Adzuki beans
- Black beans
- Chickpeas
- Mung beans, split
- Mung beans, whole
- Split peas

OILS

- Coconut oil
- Extra-virgin olive oil
- Ghee

SPICES

- Basil
- Cardamom
- Cilantro
- Coriander
- Dill
- Fennel
- Mint
- Parsley

SWEETENERS

- Jaggery
- Maple syrup
- Sucanat

Autumn Shopping List

FRUITS

- Avocados
- Bananas
- Dates
- Figs
- Grapes
- Lemons
- Mangos
- Oranges
- Papayas
- Prunes, soaked
- Raisins, soaked
- Tangerines

VEGETABLES

- Beets
- Carrots
- Okra
- Pumpkins
- Sweet potatoes
- Winter squash

GRAINS

- Amaranth
- Basmati rice
- Brown rice
- Rolled oats (dry)
- Wheat
- Wild rice

LEGUMES

- Miso
- Mung beans, split
- Mung beans, whole

NUTS AND SEEDS

- Almonds
- Brazil nuts
- Cashews
- Hazelnuts
- Pistachio
- Pumpkin seeds
- Sesame seeds
- Sunflower seeds
- Walnuts

DAIRY

- Butter
- Buttermilk
- Cheese
- Cream
- Ghee
- Kefir
- Milk, boiled
- Sour cream
- Yogurt

OILS

- Extra-virgin olive oil
- Ghee
- Sesame oil

SWEETENERS

- Honey
- Jaggery
- Maple syrup
- Molasses
- Rice syrup
- Sucanat

SPICES

- Allspice
- Anise
- Basil
- Bay leaf
- Black pepper
- Cardamom
- Cinnamon
- Cloves
- Cumin
- Dill
- Ginger
- Mustard seeds
- Nutmeg
- Paprika
- Parsley
- Rosemary
- Saffron
- Turmeric

Winter Shopping List

FRUITS

- Apples (cooked)
- Apricots
- Bananas
- Berries
- Cherries
- Dates
- Grapefruit
- Lemons
- Limes
- Mangos
- Oranges
- Papayas
- Peaches
- Prunes (soaked)
- Tangerines

VEGETABLES

- Asparagus
- Beets
- Broccoli
- Brussels sprouts
- Carrots
- Cauliflower
- Green beans
- Leafy greens (cooked)
- Okra
- Pumpkin
- Radishes
- Spinach (cooked)
- Sweet potatoes
- Turnips
- Winter squash

GRAINS

- Amaranth
- Barley
- Basmati rice
- Brown rice
- Buckwheat
- Millet
- Oats
- Quinoa
- Rye
- Seitan
- Wheat
- Wild rice

LEGUMES

- Lentils
- Miso
- Mung beans, split
- Mung beans, whole
- Navy beans
- Tofu

NUTS AND SEEDS

- Almonds
- Brazil nuts
- Cashews
- Hazelnuts
- Macadamia nuts
- Peanuts
- Pecans
- Pine nuts
- Pistachios
- Pumpkin seeds
- Sunflower seeds
- Walnuts

DAIRY

- Cottage cheese
- Cow's milk, warmed
- Ghee
- Goat's milk, warmed
- Paneer
- Sour cream

OILS

- Almond oil
- Extra-virgin olive oil
- Ghee
- Mustard oil
- Sesame oil
- Sunflower oil

SWEETENERS

- Honey
- Jaggery
- Molasses
- Spices (all spices will generally be supportive during the Winter months)
- Basil
- Black pepper
- Cayenne
- Cinnamon
- Cloves
- Coriander
- Cumin
- Fennel seed
- Fenugreek
- Ginger
- Mustard seeds
- Oregano
- Red pepper flakes
- Rosemary
- Tarragon

The Substances of Our Universe

Pratyaksha means "direct perception," and in Ayurveda it is considered the most important aspect of wisdom. The early sages of Ayurveda paid close attention to nature and identified 10 pairs of opposite properties, which they broke down and tallied up into the 20 attributes that articulate the essence of all that we experience in the material world.

The 20 Attributes

Heavy	Light
Dull	Sharp
Hot	Cold
Oily/Wet	Dry
Smooth	Rough
Dense	Liquid/Spreading
Hard	Soft
Gross	Subtle
Stable/Static	Mobile
Cloudy/Sticky	Clear

Nature evolved intelligently, with a right balance of nourishing and purifying actions. Think, for instance, about your breath. As you take in a deep inhale, you can feel its nourishment. As you exhale, long and slow, you can feel a release, a letting go. Your breath inhales the nourishment of oxygen. It exhales the toxins of carbon dioxide.

This inhale-exhale is everywhere present in nature. The earth spinning around its own axis gives us night and day. During the day, we feed ourselves on sensory input and experiences. At night our bodies rest, so we can purify and restore. Nature does this, too. With her seasons of Spring and Summer, she feeds. In Autumn she sheds, releases, and turns inward for Winter.

This primordial intelligence is also within you. Your body is perpetually adapting and adjusting to the needs of the moment, healing and purifying, nourishing, transforming, growing, shedding, recalibrating, and rebalancing.

Just to be aware of each inhale and exhale, the breath of nature flowing through you, is enough to create homeostasis, the elegant balance where all healing occurs.

I invite you to remember that you are this genius of life, and to enjoy the intelligence of nature in her food, and in you, with every sumptuous bite.

The Dirty Dozen & The Clean Fifteen

A nonprofit environmental watchdog organization called Environmental Working Group (EWG) looks at data supplied by the US Department of Agriculture (USDA) and the Food and Drug Administration (FDA) about pesticide residues. Each year it compiles a list of the best and worst pesticide loads found in commercial crops. You can use these lists to decide which fruits and vegetables to buy organic to minimize your exposure to pesticides and which produce is considered safe enough to buy conventionally. This does not mean they are pesticide-free, though, so wash these fruits and vegetables thoroughly.

These lists change every year, so make sure you look up the most recent one before you fill your shopping cart. You'll find the most recent lists, as well as a guide to pesticides in produce, at EWG.org/FoodNews.

Dirty Dozen

Apples	Nectarines	*In addition to the Dirty Dozen, the EWG added two types of produce contaminated with highly toxic organophosphate insecticides:*
Celery	Peaches	
Cherries	Spinach	
Cherry tomatoes	Strawberries	
Cucumbers	Sweet bell peppers	Kale/Collard greens
Grapes	Tomatoes	Hot peppers

Clean Fifteen

Asparagus	Eggplant	Onions
Avocados	Grapefruit	Papayas
Cabbage	Honeydew melon	Pineapples
Cantaloupe	Kiwifruits	Sweet corn
Cauliflower	Mangos	Sweet peas (frozen)

Resources

Articles

Hadhazy, Adam. "Think Twice: How the Gut's 'Second Brain' Influences Mood and Well-Being." *Scientific American*. February 12, 2010. www.scientificamerican .com/article/gut-second-brain.

Books

Bohlen, Susan Weis. *Ayurveda Beginner's Guide*. Emeryville, CA: Althea Press, 2017. An introductory guide to Ayurveda that offers a balanced mix of background information, step-by-step practices, and home remedies to help beginners start applying Ayurvedic principles right away.

Chaudhury, Kureet. *Prime: Prepare and Repair Your Body for Optimal Weight Loss*. New York: Harmony Books, 2016. An integrative neurologist and Ayurvedic practitioner explains how to sharpen the brain and smarten the gut for healing with Ayurvedic wisdom and a plan.

Frawley, David, and Ranade Subhash. *Ayurveda, Nature's Medicine*. Twin Lakes, WI: Lotus Press, 2001. From diet and herbs to Yoga and meditation, to diagnostic and treatment methods, the practices of Ayurveda are comprehensively described, emphasizing Ayurveda's roots as a spiritual science grounded in nature.

Kshirsagar, Suhas G. *The Hot Belly Diet: A 30-Day Ayurvedic Plan to Reset Your Metabolism, Lose Weight, and Restore Your Body's Natural Balance to Heal Itself*. New York: Atria Books, 2014. A total-body health plan centered on digestive balance and metabolic transformation from internationally award-winning author Dr. Suhas Kshirsagar.

Lad, Vasant. *Ayurveda: The Science of Self-Healing*. Twin Lakes, WI: Lotus Press, 1985. An Ayurvedic classic, this brief guide describes the basics of Ayurveda in a concise and straightforward manner.

Lad, Vasant. *The Complete Book of Ayurvedic Home Remedies*. New York: Harmony Books, 1999. Natural alternatives to conventional medicines and treatments with practical advice and easy-to-follow instructions from one of the Ayurvedic legends of our time.

Morningstar, Amadea. *The Ayurvedic Cookbook*. Twin Lakes, WI: Lotus Press, 1992. This classic offers mostly Indian-style recipes, with details about the doshas listed for each.

Sapolsky, Robert M. *Why Zebras Don't Get Ulcers*, 3rd ed. New York: Henry Holt & Company, 2004. By a Stanford professor of biology and neurology, this New York Times bestseller discusses the effects of prolonged stress on a range of physical and mental ailments and offers advice for controlling stress responses.

Tiwari, Bri Maya. *The Path of Practice: A Woman's Book of Ayurvedic Healing*. New York: Ballantine Books, 2001. A treasure of Ayurvedic wisdom, easy recipes, meditations, and exercises, interwoven with the author's personal stories of her clients' healing and her own journey from disease sufferer to spiritual sage.

Yarema, Thomas, Daniel Rhoda, and Johnny Branigan. *Eat Taste Heal: An Ayurvedic Cookbook for Modern Living*. Kapaa, HI: Five Elements Press, 2006. One of the first books to interpret Ayurvedic cooking for the Western palate, this book is clear and colorful, with delicious, easy-to-follow recipes.

Blogs

Joyful Belly, www.joyfulbelly.com
Created by John Immel, Joyful Belly is a great online compendium of foods and their five elements, recipes and their six tastes, and doshas and their best practices. Includes an online shop for teas and herbs.

Food: A Love Story, food-alovestory.com
My blog offers more than 200 healthy, whole-food, plant-based recipes while applying the principles of Ayurveda to the seasons, a Western sensibility, and modern lifestyles.

Vidya Living, vidyaliving.com/recipes
Vidya means "clarity, knowledge, inner wisdom." For Claire Ragazzino, vidya is where wellness begins, and she shares that beautifully in sumptuously photographed posts fusing the ancient practices of Ayurveda and Yoga with modern plant-based nutrition.

Yoga Healer, www.yogahealer.com/blog
Cate Stillman's blog delivers *Pitta* smart healing wisdom in an everyday girlfriend manner, making her Ayurvedic inspiration easy, playful, endearing, and most important of all, doable.

Hey Monica B, www.heymonicab.com/blog
A graphic designer and working mom, Monica Bloom offers up big graphics, clear writing, and pared-down methods to make Ayurveda fit a busy modern lifestyle.

Ayurvedic Suppliers

Banyan Botanicals, www.banyanbotanicals.com
A wide variety of sustainably sourced and fair-trade Ayurvedic products, along with a rich trove of information about Ayurveda, the doshas, wellness management, and daily self-care.

Maharishi Ayur-Veda Products International, www.mapi.com
Quality Ayurvedic herbal products, including herbal formulas, natural skin care products, massage oils, aroma therapy blends, teas, and spice blends, as well as articles to deepen your wisdom.

AyurFoods, www.ayurfoods.com
Ayurvedic doctor and biochemist Dr. Jay Apte created vegan, vegetarian, six-taste-balanced, whole-food, Ayurvedic meals in two- to three-serving packages that cook up in 10 minutes or less.

Ancient India, www.ancientorganics.com
A pure and delicious ghee, made by Ayurvedic devotees, sourced from organic pastured butter and prepared with strict adherence to the ancient techniques and considerations of ghee making.

Ayurvedic Clinics

Kerala Ayurveda Fremont Center, www.keralaayurveda.us/fremont
The clinical arm of Kerala Ayurveda Academy, this traditional Ayurvedic healing center balances rigor with warmth and accessibility.

Ayurvedic Healing Clinic, www.ayurvedichealing.net
A full-service Ayurvedic clinic run by leading Ayurvedic experts Drs. Manisha and Suhas Kshirsagar in Santa Cruz, California.

The Ayurvedic Institute, www.ayurveda.com
Recognized as one of the leading Ayurveda schools and Ayurvedic health spas outside of India, and led by one of America's first teachers of Ayurveda, the brilliant and beloved Dr. Vasant Lad.

Hale Pule Ayurveda, www.halepule.com
Ayurvedic treatments, classes, Yoga, meditation, Durga organic gardens, and personally designed healing with Myra Lewin and her experienced team on Kauai, Hawaii.

Vaidyagrama, www.vaidyagrama.com
An authentic healing village in South India for 21-day stays or longer. Excellent for chronic illness or deep rejuvenation.

Find a Practitioner, ayurvedanextdoor.com/directory
To find an Ayurvedic doctor, practitioner, clinic, or classes near you, check this website, which also offers articles and online courses.

Season & Dosha Recipe Index

SPRING

Amaranth Chai Porridge, 87
Apricot Tapioca Pudding, 160
Asparagus & Barley Bowl, 99
Basil Pesto, 175
Beans & Greens, 101
Berry & Peach Panzanella, 104
Breakfast Chia Pudding, 90
Breakfast Soup, 91
Cilantro Pesto, 174
Coconut Chai, 74
Creamy Quinoa, 86
Creamy Watercress Soup, 123
Curried Green Beans, 135
Fennel & Fava Bean Soup, 138–139
Ginger Broccolini, 125
Ginger, Lemon & Honey Tea, 72
Homemade Pumpkin Seed Milk, 68
Hot & Spicy Oil, 64
Mint Pea Soup, 126
Miso Soup with Asparagus, 122
Rice & Bean Hummus, 183
Simple Saag, 124
Spicy Popcorn, 162
Spinach Paneer, 100
Spring Kitchari, 98
Spring Pea Salad, 102
Spring Spice Blend, 60

SUMMER

Avocado Mash, 184
Basil Pesto, 175
Beans & Greens, 101
Berry & Peach Panzanella, 104
Borscht, 136–137
Breakfast Chia Pudding, 90
Buckwheat Pancakes, 94
Cauli Tacos, 149
Chocolate Pudding, 165
Cilantro Pesto, 174
Coconut-Mango Crumble, 169
Coconut-Mint Chutney, 177
Coconut Squash Dal, 128
Creamy Quinoa, 86
Cucumber-Mint Cooler, 78
Ginger Broccolini, 125
Healthy Hot Chocolate, 170
Homemade Almond Milk, 67
Homemade Coconut Milk, 66
Homemade Pumpkin Seed Milk, 68
Mango & Cabbage Salad, 106
Mint Pea Soup, 126
Peaches & Cream Smoothie, 79
Persian Cucumber Salad, 105
PLT Sandwiches, 156
Pumpkin Nut Bread, 95
Quesadillas, 152
Rice & Bean Hummus, 183
Rice Biryani, 132–133
Rice Pudding, 84
Roasted Vegetable Bowl, 109
Rose Fennel Tea, 77
Simple Saag, 124
Spring Pea Salad, 102
Summer Gazpacho, 127
Summer Kitchari, 103
Summer Spice Blend, 61
Sweet & Spicy Oil, 65
Thai Noodle Salad, 107
Tofu Tamari Bowl, 108
Yam Fries, 150
Yogurt-Dill Dipping Sauce, 182

AUTUMN

Amaranth Chai Porridge, 87
Autumn Kitchari, 110
Autumn Spice Blend, 62
Borscht, 136–137
Buckwheat Pancakes, 94
Carrot Halva, 168
Carrot Pickle, 185
Cauli Tacos, 149
Chocolate Pudding, 165
Cilantro Pesto, 174

Coconut Chai, 74
Coconut-Mango Crumble, 169
Crunchy Yogurt Bowl, 88
Curried Cashews, 161
Curried Green Beans, 135
Digestive Lassi, 75
Farmer's Cheese Spread, 112
Fennel & Fava Bean Soup, 138–139
Ginger-Carrot Soup, 131
Gravy & Mash, 153
Healthy Hot Chocolate, 170
Homemade Almond Milk, 67
Homemade Coconut Milk, 66
Hot & Spicy Oil, 64
Lemony Ginger Chutney, 178
Lentil Lasagna, 146–147
Nutty-Crusted Apple Pie, 166–167
Nutty Oatmeal, 85
Pistachio Rice with Tahini Yogurt, 113
Pistachio Truffles, 164
Preserved Lemons, 179
Pumpkin Nut Bread, 95
Quesadillas, 152
Rice Biryani, 132–133
Rice Pudding, 84
Roasted Roots Ecrasse, 129
Roasted Vegetable Bowl, 109
Rose Fennel Tea, 77
Rose Lassi, 76
Sesame Noodle Stir-Fry, 111
Stuffed Dates, 163
Sweet & Spicy Oil, 65
Sweet Potato Jackets, 157
Thai Noodle Salad, 107
Yam Fries, 150
Yogurt-Dill Dipping Sauce, 182

WINTER

Amaranth Chai Porridge, 87
Beans & Greens, 101
Borscht, 136–137
Breakfast Chia Pudding, 90
Breakfast Soup, 91
Buckwheat Pancakes, 94
Carrot Halva, 168
Carrot Pickle, 185

Cilantro Pesto, 174
Coconut Chai, 74
Creamy Quinoa, 86
Curried Green Beans, 135
Digestive Lassi, 75
Fennel & Fava Bean Soup, 138–139
Ginger Broccolini, 125
Ginger-Carrot Soup, 131
Ginger, Lemon & Honey Tea, 72
Gravy & Mash, 153
Healthy Hot Chocolate, 170
Homemade Coconut Milk, 66
Hot & Spicy Oil, 64
Kerala Cauliflower Stew, 117
Lentil Lasagna, 146–147
Miso Soup with Asparagus, 122
Nutty Oatmeal, 85
Preserved Lemons, 179
Pumpkin Nut Bread, 95
Quesadillas, 152
Rice Biryani, 132–133
Rice Pudding, 84
Roasted Vegetable Bowl, 109
Rose Lassi, 76
Spicy Popcorn, 162
Winter Kitchari, 114
Winter Risotto, 116
Winter Spice Blend, 63
Yam Fries, 150

YEAR-ROUND

Apple Chutney, 176
Asian Noodle Soup, 130
Basic Broth, 59
Breakfast Crêpes with Cinnamon-
    Orange Honey, 92–93
CCF Digest Tea, 73
Chapatis, 69
Cinnamon-Honey Syrup, 186
Cucumber Raita, 180
Deep-Sleep Tonic, 81
Delicious Dal, 115
Easy Homemade Jam, 171
Flatbread Pizza, 151
Ghee, 58
Golden Milk, 80

Healing Kanji, 141
Kitchari "Burgers," 144
Mung Bean Soup, 120
Pasta al Pesto, 145
Pho Soup, 134
Pumpkin Seed Butter, 181
Restorative Roots & Shoots Broth, 121
Rice & Bean Burritos, 148
Seasonal Fruit Compote, 89
Seasonal Vegetable Purée, 140
Whole-Skillet Hash Browns, 154–155

KAPHA

Amaranth Chai Porridge, 87
Apple Chutney, 176
Apricot Tapioca Pudding, 160
Asparagus & Barley Bowl, 99
Basic Broth, 59
Basil Pesto, 175
Beans & Greens, 101
Berry & Peach Panzanella, 104
Breakfast Chia Pudding, 90
Breakfast Crêpes with Cinnamon-
     Orange Honey, 92–93
Breakfast Soup, 91
Buckwheat Pancakes, 94
CCF Digest Tea, 73
Chapatis, 69
Chocolate Pudding, 165
Cilantro Pesto, 174
Cinnamon-Honey Syrup, 186
Coconut Chai, 74
Creamy Quinoa, 86
Creamy Watercress Soup, 123
Cucumber Raita, 180
Curried Green Beans, 135
Delicious Dal, 115
Easy Homemade Jam, 171
Fennel & Fava Bean Soup, 138–139
Flatbread Pizza, 151
Ghee, 58
Ginger Broccolini, 125
Ginger-Carrot Soup, 131
Ginger, Lemon & Honey Tea, 72
Golden Milk, 80
Homemade Coconut Milk, 66

Homemade Pumpkin Seed Milk, 68
Hot & Spicy Oil, 64
Kerala Cauliflower Stew, 117
Kitchari "Burgers," 144
Lentil Lasagna, 146–147
Mango & Cabbage Salad, 106
Mint Pea Soup, 126
Miso Soup with Asparagus, 122
Mung Bean Soup, 120
Nutty-Crusted Apple Pie, 166–167
Pasta al Pesto, 145
Peaches & Cream Smoothie, 79
Preserved Lemons, 179
Pumpkin Seed Butter, 181
Rice & Bean Burritos, 148
Rice & Bean Hummus, 183
Rice Biryani, 132–133
Rice Pudding, 84
Roasted Vegetable Bowl, 109
Seasonal Fruit Compote, 89
Seasonal Vegetable Purée, 140
Simple Saag, 124
Spicy Popcorn, 162
Spinach Paneer, 100
Spring Kitchari, 98
Spring Pea Salad, 102
Spring Spice Blend, 60
Tofu Tamari Bowl, 108
Whole-Skillet Hash Browns, 154–155
Winter Kitchari, 114
Winter Spice Blend, 63

PITTA

Apple Chutney, 176
Asian Noodle Soup, 130
Asparagus & Barley Bowl, 99
Avocado Mash, 184
Basic Broth, 59
Basil Pesto, 175
Beans & Greens, 101
Berry & Peach Panzanella, 104
Borscht, 136–137
Breakfast Chia Pudding, 90
Breakfast Crêpes with
     Cinnamon-Orange Honey, 92–93
Breakfast Soup, 91

Buckwheat Pancakes, 94
Cauli Tacos, 149
CCF Digest Tea, 73
Chapatis, 69
Chocolate Pudding, 165
Cilantro Pesto, 174
Coconut Chai, 74
Coconut-Mango Crumble, 169
Coconut-Mint Chutney, 177
Coconut Squash Dal, 128
Creamy Quinoa, 86
Creamy Watercress Soup, 123
Cucumber-Mint Cooler, 78
Cucumber Raita, 180
Curried Green Beans, 135
Deep-Sleep Tonic, 81
Delicious Dal, 115
Easy Homemade Jam, 171
Fennel & Fava Bean Soup, 138–139
Flatbread Pizza, 151
Ghee, 58
Ginger Broccolini, 125
Ginger-Carrot Soup, 131
Golden Milk, 80
Healing Kanji, 141
Healthy Hot Chocolate, 170
Homemade Almond Milk, 67
Homemade Coconut Milk, 66
Homemade Pumpkin Seed Milk, 68
Kerala Cauliflower Stew, 117
Kitchari "Burgers," 144
Lentil Lasagna, 146–147
Mango & Cabbage Salad, 106
Mint Pea Soup, 126
Miso Soup with Asparagus, 122
Mung Bean Soup, 120
Nutty-Crusted Apple Pie, 166–167
Nutty Oatmeal, 85
Pasta al Pesto, 145
Peaches & Cream Smoothie, 79
Persian Cucumber Salad, 105
Pistachio Truffles, 164
PLT Sandwiches, 156
Preserved Lemons, 179
Pumpkin Nut Bread, 95
Pumpkin Seed Butter, 181

Quesadillas, 152
Rice & Bean Burritos, 148
Rice & Bean Hummus, 183
Rice Biryani, 132–133
Rice Pudding, 84
Roasted Roots Ecrasse, 129
Roasted Vegetable Bowl, 109
Rose Fennel Tea, 77
Rose Lassi, 76
Seasonal Fruit Compote, 89
Seasonal Vegetable Purée, 140
Sesame Noodle Stir-Fry, 111
Simple Saag, 124
Spinach Paneer, 100
Spring Pea Salad, 102
Summer Gazpacho, 127
Summer Kitchari, 103
Summer Spice Blend, 61
Sweet & Spicy Oil, 65
Sweet Potato Jackets, 157
Thai Noodle Salad, 107
Tofu Tamari Bowl, 108
Whole-Skillet Hash Browns, 154–155
Winter Risotto, 116
Yam Fries, 150
Yogurt-Dill Dipping Sauce, 182

VATA

Amaranth Chai Porridge, 87
Apple Chutney, 176
Asian Noodle Soup, 130
Autumn Kitchari, 110
Autumn Spice Blend, 62
Avocado Mash, 184
Basic Broth, 59
Basil Pesto, 175
Berry & Peach Panzanella, 104
Borscht, 136–137
Breakfast Chia Pudding, 90
Breakfast Crêpes with Cinnamon-
    Orange Honey, 92–93
Breakfast Soup, 91
Buckwheat Pancakes, 94
Carrot Halva, 168
Carrot Pickle, 185
Cauli Tacos, 149

CCF Digest Tea, 73
Chapatis, 69
Chocolate Pudding, 165
Coconut Chai, 74
Coconut-Mango Crumble, 169
Coconut-Mint Chutney, 177
Creamy Watercress Soup, 123
Crunchy Yogurt Bowl, 88
Cucumber Raita, 180
Curried Cashews, 161
Curried Green Beans, 135
Deep-Sleep Tonic, 81
Delicious Dal, 115
Digestive Lassi, 75
Easy Homemade Jam, 171
Farmer's Cheese Spread, 112
Fennel & Fava Bean Soup, 138–139
Flatbread Pizza, 151
Ghee, 58
Ginger-Carrot Soup, 131
Ginger, Lemon & Honey Tea, 72
Golden Milk, 80
Gravy & Mash, 153
Healing Kanji, 141
Healthy Hot Chocolate, 170
Homemade Almond Milk, 67
Homemade Coconut Milk, 66
Hot & Spicy Oil, 64
Kerala Cauliflower Stew, 117
Kitchari "Burgers," 144
Lemony Ginger Chutney, 178
Lentil Lasagna, 146–147
Mango & Cabbage Salad, 106
Miso Soup with Asparagus, 122
Mung Bean Soup, 120
Nutty-Crusted Apple Pie, 166–167

Nutty Oatmeal, 85
Pasta al Pesto, 145
Peaches & Cream Smoothie, 79
Pho Soup, 134
Pistachio Rice with Tahini Yogurt, 113
Pistachio Truffles, 164
PLT Sandwiches, 156
Preserved Lemons, 179
Pumpkin Nut Bread, 95
Pumpkin Seed Butter, 181
Quesadillas, 152
Restorative Roots & Shoots Broth, 121
Rice & Bean Burritos, 148
Rice Biryani, 132–133
Rice Pudding, 84
Roasted Roots Ecrasse, 129
Roasted Vegetable Bowl, 109
Rose Fennel Tea, 77
Rose Lassi, 76
Seasonal Fruit Compote, 89
Seasonal Vegetable Purée, 140
Sesame Noodle Stir-Fry, 111
Simple Saag, 124
Spinach Paneer, 100
Spring Pea Salad, 102
Stuffed Dates, 163
Sweet & Spicy Oil, 65
Sweet Potato Jackets, 157
Thai Noodle Salad, 107
Tofu Tamari Bowl, 108
Whole-Skillet Hash Browns, 154–155
Winter Kitchari, 114
Winter Risotto, 116
Winter Spice Blend, 63
Yam Fries, 150
Yogurt-Dill Dipping Sauce, 182

Recipe Index

A

Amaranth Chai Porridge, 87
Apple Chutney, 176
Apricot Tapioca Pudding, 160
Asian Noodle Soup, 130
Asparagus & Barley Bowl, 99
Autumn Kitchari, 110
Autumn Spice Blend, 62
Avocado Mash, 184

B

Basic Broth, 59
Basil Pesto, 175
Beans & Greens, 101
Berry & Peach Panzanella, 104
Borscht, 136–137
Breakfast Chia Pudding, 90
Breakfast Crêpes with
    Cinnamon-Orange Honey, 92–93
Breakfast Soup, 91
Buckwheat Pancakes, 94

C

Carrot Halva, 168
Carrot Pickle, 185
Cauli Tacos, 149
CCF Digest Tea, 73
Chapatis, 69
Chocolate Pudding, 165
Cilantro Pesto, 174
Cinnamon-Honey Syrup, 186
Coconut Chai, 74
Coconut-Mango Crumble, 169
Coconut-Mint Chutney, 177
Coconut Squash Dal, 128
Creamy Quinoa, 86
Creamy Watercress Soup, 123
Crunchy Yogurt Bowl, 88
Cucumber-Mint Cooler, 78
Cucumber Raita, 180
Curried Cashews, 161
Curried Green Beans, 135

D

Deep-Sleep Tonic, 81
Delicious Dal, 115
Digestive Lassi, 75

E

Easy Homemade Jam, 171

F

Farmer's Cheese Spread, 112
Fennel & Fava Bean Soup, 138–139
Flatbread Pizza, 151

G

Ghee, 58
Ginger Broccolini, 125
Ginger-Carrot Soup, 131
Ginger, Lemon & Honey Tea, 72
Golden Milk, 80
Gravy & Mash, 153

H

Healing Kanji, 141
Healthy Hot Chocolate, 170
Homemade Almond Milk, 67
Homemade Coconut Milk, 66
Homemade Pumpkin Seed Milk, 68
Hot & Spicy Oil, 64

K

Kerala Cauliflower Stew, 117
Kitchari "Burgers," 144

L

Lemony Ginger Chutney, 178
Lentil Lasagna, 146–147

M

Mango & Cabbage Salad, 106
Mint Pea Soup, 126

Miso Soup with Asparagus, 122
Mung Bean Soup, 120

N

Nutty-Crusted Apple Pie, 166–167
Nutty Oatmeal, 85

P

Pasta al Pesto, 145
Peaches & Cream Smoothie, 79
Persian Cucumber Salad, 105
Pho Soup, 134
Pistachio Rice with Tahini Yogurt, 113
Pistachio Truffles, 164
PLT Sandwiches, 156
Preserved Lemons, 179
Pumpkin Nut Bread, 95
Pumpkin Seed Butter, 181

Q

Quesadillas, 152

R

Restorative Roots & Shoots Broth, 121
Rice & Bean Burritos, 148
Rice & Bean Hummus, 183
Rice Biryani, 132–133
Rice Pudding, 84
Roasted Roots Ecrasse, 129
Roasted Vegetable Bowl, 109
Rose Fennel Tea, 77
Rose Lassi, 76

S

Seasonal Fruit Compote, 89
Seasonal Vegetable Purée, 140
Sesame Noodle Stir-Fry, 111
Simple Saag, 124
Spicy Popcorn, 162
Spinach Paneer, 100
Spring Kitchari, 98
Spring Pea Salad, 102
Spring Spice Blend, 60
Stuffed Dates, 163
Summer Gazpacho, 127
Summer Kitchari, 103
Summer Spice Blend, 61
Sweet & Spicy Oil, 65
Sweet Potato Jackets, 157

T

Thai Noodle Salad, 107
Tofu Tamari Bowl, 108

W

Whole-Skillet Hash Browns, 154–155
Winter Kitchari, 114
Winter Risotto, 116
Winter Spice Blend, 63

Y

Yam Fries, 150
Yogurt-Dill Dipping Sauce, 182

Index

A

Age, 16
Agni, 21, 26–28, 37, 51
Ahimsa, 36
Almond butter
    Nutty-Crusted Apple Pie, 166–167
    Sesame Noodle Stir-Fry, 111
    Stuffed Dates, 163
Almond flour
    Pumpkin Nut Bread, 95
Ama, 27–28
Amaranth
    Amaranth Chai Porridge, 87
Anjali, 38
Apples
    Amaranth Chai Porridge, 87
    Apple Chutney, 176
    Nutty-Crusted Apple Pie, 166–167
    Peaches & Cream Smoothie, 79
    Pumpkin Nut Bread, 95
    Seasonal Fruit Compote, 89
Apricots
    Apricot Tapioca Pudding, 160
Arugula
    Berry & Peach Panzanella, 104
    Persian Cucumber Salad, 105
Ashtanga Hridayam, 14
Asparagus
    Asparagus & Barley Bowl, 99
    Miso Soup with Asparagus, 122
Astringent tastes, 31
Autumn
    about, 15, 19
    meal plan, 46
    shopping list, 200
    tastes and qualities, 34
Avocados
    Avocado Mash, 184
    Chocolate Pudding, 165
    Mango & Cabbage Salad, 106
    Rice & Bean Burritos, 148
    Summer Gazpacho, 127

Awareness, 6, 50–51
Ayurveda. See also Foods
    guiding principles in, 18–21, 23
    healthy diet principles, 35
    history of, 4
    modalities, 5
    and modern life, 4–5
    role of food in, 26
    and self-inquiry, 6
    and the universal
        elements, 8–18, 202
    vital essences of, 7–8

B

Balance, 4, 7–8, 19–20, 38. See
    also Doshas
Barley
    Asparagus & Barley Bowl, 99
Basil
    Autumn Kitchari, 110
    Basil Pesto, 175
    Pasta al Pesto, 145
    Peaches & Cream Smoothie, 79
    Pistachio Truffles, 164
    Spring Kitchari, 98
Beets
    Borscht, 136–137
    Carrot Pickle, 185
    Restorative Roots & Shoots
        Broth, 121
Berries
    Berry & Peach Panzanella, 104
    Easy Homemade Jam, 171
    Seasonal Fruit Compote, 89
Beverages. See also Teas
    Cucumber-Mint Cooler, 78
    Deep-Sleep Tonic, 81
    Digestive Lassi, 75
    Golden Milk, 80
    Peaches & Cream Smoothie, 79
    Rose Lassi, 76
Bitter tastes, 31

Blake, William, 197
Bok choy
    Pho Soup, 134
    Sesame Noodle Stir-Fry, 111
Bowls
    Asparagus & Barley Bowl, 99
    Crunchy Yogurt Bowl, 88
    Roasted Vegetable Bowl, 109
    Tofu Tamari Bowl, 108
Breathing, 6
Broccolini
    Ginger Broccolini, 125
Buckwheat flour
    Buckwheat Pancakes, 94

C

Cabbage. See also Kimchi; Sauerkraut
    Mango & Cabbage Salad, 106
    Spring Pea Salad, 102
Cacao powder
    Chocolate Pudding, 165
    Healthy Hot Chocolate, 170
Carrots
    Basic Broth, 59
    Breakfast Soup, 91
    Carrot Halva, 168
    Carrot Pickle, 185
    Cucumber Raita, 180
    Ginger-Carrot Soup, 131
    Kerala Cauliflower Stew, 117
    Rice Biryani, 132-133
    Sesame Noodle Stir-Fry, 111
Cauliflower
    Cauli Tacos, 149
    Kerala Cauliflower Stew, 117
Celery
    Basic Broth, 59
    Fennel & Fava Bean Soup, 138-139
    Restorative Roots & Shoots
        Broth, 121
    Winter Risotto, 116
Charaka Samhita, 36
Chard
    Asparagus & Barley Bowl, 99
Cherries
    Breakfast Chia Pudding, 90

Chia seeds
    Breakfast Chia Pudding, 90
    Nutty-Crusted Apple
        Pie, 166-167
    Whole-Skillet Hash
        Browns, 154-155
Cilantro
    Apple Chutney, 176
    Cilantro Pesto, 174
    Cucumber Raita, 180
    Persian Cucumber Salad, 105
    Summer Kitchari, 103
    Thai Noodle Salad, 107
Coconut
    Coconut-Mango Crumble, 169
    Coconut-Mint Chutney, 177
    Creamy Quinoa, 86
    Homemade Coconut Milk, 66
    PLT Sandwiches, 156
    Pumpkin Nut Bread, 95
    Summer Kitchari, 103
Cohesion. See Ojas
Consciousness, 4
Cucumbers
    Cucumber-Mint Cooler, 78
    Cucumber Raita, 180
    Persian Cucumber Salad, 105
    Summer Gazpacho, 127
Curry leaves
    Curried Cashews, 161

D

Dairy products, 30, 48. See also
        Milk; Yogurt
Dandelion leaves
    Berry & Peach Panzanella, 104
Dates
    Deep-Sleep Tonic, 81
    Homemade Almond Milk, 67
    Nutty-Crusted Apple
        Pie, 166-167
    Pistachio Truffles, 164
    Rice Pudding, 84
    Stuffed Dates, 163
Digestion, 26-28, 37, 51
Digestive system, 21

Dill
    Persian Cucumber Salad, 105
    Sweet Potato Jackets, 157
    Yogurt-Dill Dipping Sauce, 182
Doshas. See also specific
    about, 8–9, 20–21
    balancing, 12–14, 22, 33–34, 189
    determining predominant, 10–12
    dual, 13–14, 195–196
    examining your doshic
      environment, 42–43
    foods for, 32
    qualities of, 14
Dulse
    Breakfast Soup, 91
    Summer Kitchari, 103
Dynamism. See Prana

E

Eating, 38–39
Empowerment, 5
Energy, 19
Equilibrium, 4. See also Balance
Equipment, 50

F

Fava beans
    Fennel & Fava Bean Soup, 138–139
Fennel
    Fennel & Fava Bean Soup, 138–139
Fenugreek
    Simple Saag, 124
Flax eggs, 94
Flaxseed
    Amaranth Chai Porridge, 87
    Creamy Quinoa, 86
    Crunchy Yogurt Bowl, 88
    Pumpkin Nut Bread, 95
    Whole-Skillet Hash Browns, 154–155
Foods
    to avoid, 35–36
    and digestion, 26–28, 37, 51
    good combining, 28
    gunas, 28, 30
    healthy diet principles, 35

    healthy routines, 38–39
    pantry staples, 48, 197
    role of in Ayurveda, 26
    six tastes of, 30–31, 33
    20 qualities/attributes and, 17
Fruits, 27, 48. See also specific

G

Ginger
    Asian Noodle Soup, 130
    Asparagus & Barley Bowl, 99
    Beans & Greens, 101
    Borscht, 136–137
    Carrot Pickle, 185
    Cinnamon-Honey Syrup, 186
    Coconut-Mint Chutney, 177
    Creamy Watercress Soup, 123
    Curried Green Beans, 135
    Ginger Broccolini, 125
    Ginger-Carrot Soup, 131
    Ginger, Lemon & Honey Tea, 72
    Lemony Ginger Chutney, 178
    Mango & Cabbage Salad, 106
    Miso Soup with Asparagus, 122
    Mung Bean Soup, 120
    Sesame Noodle Stir-Fry, 111
    Simple Saag, 124
    Spring Pea Salad, 102
Grains, 30. See also specific
Green beans
    Curried Green Beans, 135
    Kerala Cauliflower Stew, 117
    Persian Cucumber Salad, 105
    Rice Biryani, 132–133
Gunas, 28, 30

H

Herbs. See also specific
    Beans & Greens, 101
    Fennel & Fava Bean Soup, 138–139
    Ginger-Carrot Soup, 131
    Summer Gazpacho, 127
    Winter Kitchari, 114
Hippocrates, 25
Homeostasis, 4. See also Balance

I

Individuality, 5, 7–8
Inertia, 20

J

Jaggery, 35–36

K

Kapha
    about, 9, 12–14, 193
    balancing, 22, 33–34
    dietary recommendations
      for, 193–194
    foods for, 17, 32
    lifestyle, 194
    seasons and, 15
    time and, 16
Kellogg, John Harvey, 3
Kimchi
    Pho Soup, 134
Kitchen Remedy recipes
    about, 55
    Asparagus & Barley Bowl, 99
    Autumn Kitchari, 110
    Autumn Spice Blend, 62
    Basil Pesto, 175
    Borscht, 136–137
    Carrot Pickle, 185
    CCF Digest Tea, 73
    Cilantro Pesto, 174
    Cinnamon-Honey Syrup, 186
    Coconut Chai, 74
    Coconut Squash Dal, 128
    Cucumber-Mint Cooler, 78
    Deep-Sleep Tonic, 81
    Digestive Lassi, 75
    Ginger Broccolini, 125
    Ginger-Carrot Soup, 131
    Ginger, Lemon & Honey Tea, 72
    Golden Milk, 80
    Healing Kanji, 141
    Kitchari "Burgers," 144
    Miso Soup with Asparagus, 122
    Mung Bean Soup, 120
    Peaches & Cream Smoothie, 79
    Pho Soup, 134
    Preserved Lemons, 179
    Restorative Roots & Shoots
      Broth, 121
    Roasted Roots Ecrasse, 129
    Rose Fennel Tea, 77
    Rose Lassi, 76
    Spring Kitchari, 98
    Spring Spice Blend, 60
    Summer Kitchari, 103
    Summer Spice Blend, 61
    Winter Spice Blend, 63
Kitchens, 41, 50
Kombu
    Autumn Kitchari, 110
    Seasonal Vegetable Purée, 140

L

Leafy greens. *See also specific*
    Beans & Greens, 101
    Coconut Squash Dal, 128
    Mung Bean Soup, 120
    Seasonal Vegetable Purée, 140
    Winter Risotto, 116
Legumes, 30. *See also specific*
Lemons, lemon juice, and zest
    Apple Chutney, 176
    Apricot Tapioca Pudding, 160
    Berry & Peach Panzanella, 104
    Cilantro Pesto, 174
    Cinnamon-Honey Syrup, 186
    Easy Homemade Jam, 171
    Fennel & Fava Bean Soup, 138–139
    Ginger Broccolini, 125
    Ginger-Carrot Soup, 131
    Ginger, Lemon & Honey Tea, 72
    Lemony Ginger Chutney, 178
    Lentil Lasagna, 146–147
    Nutty-Crusted Apple Pie, 166–167
    Pasta al Pesto, 145
    Pistachio Rice with Tahini
      Yogurt, 113
    Preserved Lemons, 179
    Rice & Bean Hummus, 183
    Roasted Vegetable Bowl, 109
    as a salt substitute, 36

Lemons, lemon juice,
    and zest (continued)
    Simple Saag, 124
    Spinach Paneer, 100
    Spring Pea Salad, 102
    Winter Risotto, 116
Lentils
    Lentil Lasagna, 146–147
Lettuce
    Persian Cucumber Salad, 105
    PLT Sandwiches, 156
Lifetime, 16
Like increases like, 19–20
Limes, lime juice, and zest
    Avocado Mash, 184
    Cauli Tacos, 149
    Coconut-Mango Crumble, 169
    Coconut-Mint Chutney, 177
    Cucumber-Mint Cooler, 78
    Mango & Cabbage Salad, 106
    Persian Cucumber Salad, 105
    Pho Soup, 134
    Rice & Bean Burritos, 148
    Summer Gazpacho, 127
    Yogurt-Dill Dipping Sauce, 182
Love, 41, 50–51

M

Mangos
    Coconut-Mango Crumble, 169
    Mango & Cabbage Salad, 106
Meal planning, 43–47
Meat, 36
Milk
    Buckwheat Pancakes, 94
    Carrot Halva, 168
    Deep-Sleep Tonic, 81
    Golden Milk, 80
    Spinach Paneer, 100
Mind-body connection, 23, 39
Mint
    Autumn Kitchari, 110
    Berry & Peach Panzanella, 104
    Coconut-Mint Chutney, 177
    Cucumber-Mint Cooler, 78
    Mango & Cabbage Salad, 106

Mint Pea Soup, 126
Persian Cucumber Salad, 105
Pistachio Rice with Tahini
    Yogurt, 113
PLT Sandwiches, 156
Rose Fennel Tea, 77
Summer Gazpacho, 127
Summer Kitchari, 103
Miso
    Miso Soup with Asparagus, 122
Mung beans
    Autumn Kitchari, 110
    Beans & Greens, 101
    Breakfast Crêpes with
        Cinnamon-Orange Honey, 92–93
    Coconut Squash Dal, 128
    Delicious Dal, 115
    Mung Bean Soup, 120
    Pho Soup, 134
    Spring Kitchari, 98
    Summer Kitchari, 103
    Winter Kitchari, 114
Mustard greens
    Simple Saag, 124

N

Nature, 18
Newton's laws, 20
Noodles, rice
    Asian Noodle Soup, 130
    Pasta al Pesto, 145
    Pho Soup, 134
    Thai Noodle Salad, 107
Noodles, soba
    Sesame Noodle Stir-Fry, 111
Nuts
    Basil Pesto, 175
    Carrot Halva, 168
    Curried Cashews, 161
    Curried Green Beans, 135
    Deep-Sleep Tonic, 81
    Homemade Almond Milk, 67
    Nutty-Crusted Apple Pie, 166–167
    Nutty Oatmeal, 85
    Pistachio Rice with Tahini
        Yogurt, 113

Pistachio Truffles, 164
Pumpkin Nut Bread, 95
Rice Biryani, 132–133
Thai Noodle Salad, 107

O

Oats
Nutty Oatmeal, 85
Ojas, 7–8, 8–9, 21, 81. See also Kapha
One Pot recipes
about, 55
Amaranth Chai Porridge, 87
Asparagus & Barley Bowl, 99
Autumn Kitchari, 110
Basic Broth, 59
Beans & Greens, 101
Carrot Halva, 168
Coconut Squash Dal, 128
Creamy Quinoa, 86
Fennel & Fava Bean Soup, 138–139
Ghee, 58
Gravy & Mash, 153
Healing Kanji, 141
Healthy Hot Chocolate, 170
Hot & Spicy Oil, 64
Kerala Cauliflower Stew, 117
Mung Bean Soup, 120
Pasta al Pesto, 145
Pho Soup, 134
Restorative Roots & Shoots
Broth, 121
Rice Pudding, 84
Spring Kitchari, 98
Summer Kitchari, 103
Sweet & Spicy Oil, 65
Tofu Tamari Bowl, 108
Winter Risotto, 116
Onions
Basic Broth, 59
Breakfast Soup, 91
Opposites, attraction of, 19–20
Oranges, orange juice, and zest
Berry & Peach Panzanella, 104
Breakfast Crêpes with
Cinnamon-Orange Honey, 92–93
Pistachio Truffles, 164

Seasonal Fruit Compote, 89
Whole-Skillet Hash Browns, 154–155

P

Pantry staples
Autumn Spice Blend, 62
Basic Broth, 59
Chapatis, 69
Ghee, 58
Homemade Almond Milk, 67
Homemade Coconut Milk, 66
Homemade Pumpkin Seed Milk, 68
Hot & Spicy Oil, 64
shopping list, 48, 197
Spring Spice Blend, 60
Summer Spice Blend, 61
Sweet & Spicy Oil, 65
Winter Spice Blend, 63
Parsley
Curried Green Beans, 135
Mint Pea Soup, 126
Pistachio Rice with Tahini
Yogurt, 113
Peaches
Berry & Peach Panzanella, 104
Peaches & Cream Smoothie, 79
Pears
Seasonal Fruit Compote, 89
Peas
Mint Pea Soup, 126
Perception, 4, 6
Pitta
about, 9, 12–14, 191
balancing, 22, 33–34
dietary recommendations
for, 191–192
foods for, 17, 32
lifestyle, 192–193
seasons and, 15
time and, 16
Pitta-Kapha (PK), 13–14, 196
Popcorn
Spicy Popcorn, 162
Prajnaparadha, 20
Prana, 7–8, 8–9, 21. See also Vata
Pratyaksha, 202

Produce. *See Fruits; Vegetables*
Proteins, 27
Psyllium husks
Easy Homemade Jam, 171
Kitchari "Burgers," 144
Pumpkin Nut Bread, 95
Pumpkin
Pumpkin Nut Bread, 95
Pumpkin seeds
Beans & Greens, 101
Cilantro Pesto, 174
Crunchy Yogurt Bowl, 88
Homemade Pumpkin Seed Milk, 68
Mango & Cabbage Salad, 106
Mint Pea Soup, 126
Nutty Oatmeal, 85
PLT Sandwiches, 156
Pumpkin Seed Butter, 181
Pungent tastes, 31

Q

Quinoa
Creamy Quinoa, 86
Persian Cucumber Salad, 105

R

Radiance. *See Tejas*
Radishes. *See also Kimchi*
Restorative Roots & Shoots
Broth, 121
Spring Pea Salad, 102
Raisins
Carrot Halva, 168
Pumpkin Nut Bread, 95
Rice Biryani, 132–133
Rice Pudding, 84
Rajas, 28, 30
Recipes, about, 53–55
Red (color), 41
Rice
Autumn Kitchari, 110
Breakfast Crêpes with
Cinnamon-Orange Honey, 92–93
Healing Kanji, 141
Pistachio Rice with Tahini
Yogurt, 113

Rice Biryani, 132–133
Rice Pudding, 84
Spring Kitchari, 98
Summer Kitchari, 103
Winter Kitchari, 114
Winter Risotto, 116
Root medicine, 4–5

S

Salads
Mango & Cabbage Salad, 106
Persian Cucumber Salad, 105
Spring Pea Salad, 102
Thai Noodle Salad, 107
Salt, 36
Salty tastes, 31
Sattva, 28, 30, 35
Sauerkraut
Borscht, 136–137
Seasons, 15, 18–19, 33–34.
See also specific
shopping lists, 198–201
Seeds. *See specific*
Self-inquiry, 6
Senses, 6
Sesame seeds
Asian Noodle Soup, 130
Sesame Noodle Stir-Fry, 111
Tofu Tamari Bowl, 108
Winter Kitchari, 114
Shallots
Gravy & Mash, 153
Lentil Lasagna, 146–147
Shamanism, 4
Shopping, 48
seasonal lists, 198–201
Snap peas
Spring Pea Salad, 102
Tofu Tamari Bowl, 108
Snow peas
Thai Noodle Salad, 107
Soups and stews
Asian Noodle Soup, 130
Borscht, 136–137
Creamy Watercress Soup, 123
Fennel & Fava Bean Soup, 138–139

Ginger-Carrot Soup, 131
Healing Kanji, 141
Kerala Cauliflower Stew, 117
Mint Pea Soup, 126
Miso Soup with Asparagus, 122
Mung Bean Soup, 120
Pho Soup, 134
Restorative Roots & Shoots
    Broth, 121
Summer Gazpacho, 127
Sour tastes, 31
Spices. *See also specific*
about, 36, 43, 48, 51, 73
Autumn Spice Blend, 62
Spring Spice Blend, 60
Summer Spice Blend, 61
Winter Spice Blend, 63
Spinach
Asian Noodle Soup, 130
Creamy Watercress Soup, 123
Pasta al Pesto, 145
Simple Saag, 124
Spinach Paneer, 100
Spring
about, 15, 19
meal plan, 44
shopping list, 198
tastes and qualities, 34
Squash. *See also Zucchini*
Coconut Squash Dal, 128
Stress, 21, 23
Sugar, 35–36
Summer
about, 15, 18
meal plan, 45
shopping list, 199
tastes and qualities, 34
Sunflower seeds
Crunchy Yogurt Bowl, 88
Pumpkin Seed Butter, 181
Sweet potatoes
Borscht, 136–137
Sweet Potato Jackets, 157
Whole-Skillet Hash
    Browns, 154–155
Sweet tastes, 31

T

Tahini
Pistachio Rice with Tahini
    Yogurt, 113
Rice & Bean Hummus, 183
Taittiriya Upanishad, 26, 41
Tamari
Asian Noodle Soup, 130
Asparagus & Barley Bowl, 99
Autumn Kitchari, 110
Coconut Squash Dal, 128
Curried Green Beans, 135
Gravy & Mash, 153
Miso Soup with Asparagus, 122
PLT Sandwiches, 156
Sesame Noodle Stir-Fry, 111
Tofu Tamari Bowl, 108
Winter Kitchari, 114
Tamas, 28, 30
Tapioca pearls
Apricot Tapioca Pudding, 160
Teas
about, 51
CCF Digest Tea, 73
Coconut Chai, 74
Ginger, Lemon & Honey Tea, 72
Rose Fennel Tea, 77
Tejas, 7–8, 8–9, 21. *See also Pitta*
30 Minutes or Less recipes
about, 55
Amaranth Chai Porridge, 87
Apple Chutney, 176
Apricot Tapioca Pudding, 160
Asian Noodle Soup, 130
Autumn Spice Blend, 62
Avocado Mash, 184
Basil Pesto, 175
Breakfast Chia Pudding, 90
Breakfast Crêpes with
    Cinnamon-Orange Honey, 92–93
Buckwheat Pancakes, 94
Cauli Tacos, 149
CCF Digest Tea, 73
Chapatis, 69
Chocolate Pudding, 165
Cilantro Pesto, 174

30 Minutes or Less recipes (continued)
    Coconut Chai, 74
    Coconut Squash Dal, 128
    Creamy Quinoa, 86
    Creamy Watercress Soup, 123
    Crunchy Yogurt Bowl, 88
    Cucumber-Mint Cooler, 78
    Cucumber Raita, 180
    Curried Cashews, 161
    Curried Green Beans, 135
    Deep-Sleep Tonic, 81
    Delicious Dal, 115
    Digestive Lassi, 75
    Easy Homemade Jam, 171
    Flatbread Pizza, 151
    Ghee, 58
    Ginger Broccolini, 125
    Ginger-Carrot Soup, 131
    Ginger, Lemon & Honey Tea, 72
    Golden Milk, 80
    Gravy & Mash, 153
    Healthy Hot Chocolate, 170
    Homemade Almond Milk, 67
    Homemade Coconut Milk, 66
    Homemade Pumpkin
      Seed Milk, 68
    Hot & Spicy Oil, 64
    Kerala Cauliflower Stew, 117
    Kitchari "Burgers," 144
    Lemony Ginger Chutney, 178
    Mint Pea Soup, 126
    Miso Soup with Asparagus, 122
    Nutty Oatmeal, 85
    Pasta al Pesto, 145
    Peaches & Cream Smoothie, 79
    Persian Cucumber Salad, 105
    Pho Soup, 134
    Pistachio Rice with Tahini
      Yogurt, 113
    PLT Sandwiches, 156
    Quesadillas, 152
    Restorative Roots & Shoots
      Broth, 121
    Rice & Bean Burritos, 148
    Rice & Bean Hummus, 183
    Roasted Vegetable Bowl, 109
    Rose Fennel Tea, 77
    Rose Lassi, 76
    Seasonal Fruit Compote, 89
    Seasonal Vegetable Purée, 140
    Sesame Noodle Stir-Fry, 111
    Simple Saag, 124
    Spicy Popcorn, 162
    Spinach Paneer, 100
    Spring Pea Salad, 102
    Spring Spice Blend, 60
    Stuffed Dates, 163
    Summer Gazpacho, 127
    Summer Spice Blend, 61
    Sweet & Spicy Oil, 65
    Thai Noodle Salad, 107
    Tofu Tamari Bowl, 108
    Winter Risotto, 116
    Winter Spice Blend, 63
    Yogurt-Dill Dipping Sauce, 182
Time, of day, 16
Timing, of meals, 39
Tofu
    Miso Soup with Asparagus, 122
    Tofu Tamari Bowl, 108
Tomatoes
    Lentil Lasagna, 146–147
    PLT Sandwiches, 156
    Rice & Bean Burritos, 148
    Summer Gazpacho, 127
Tools, 50
Toxins, 27–28
Tri-doshic, 13–14, 196
20 qualities/attributes, 202
    and food, 17

U

Universal elements
    about, 8
    doshas, 8–14
    and food, 17
    seasons, 15
    time, 16
    20 qualities/attributes, 17, 202

V

Vata
about, 9, 12–14, 189
balancing, 22, 33–34
dietary recommendations for, 190
foods for, 17, 32
lifestyle, 191
seasons and, 15
time and, 16
Vata-Kapha (VK), 13–14, 195–196
Vata-Pitta (VP), 13–14, 195
Vata-Pitta-Kapha (VPK), 13–14, 196
Vegetables, 30, 48. See also specific
Autumn Kitchari, 110
Roasted Roots Ecrasse, 129
Roasted Vegetable Bowl, 109
Seasonal Vegetable Purée, 140
Spring Kitchari, 98
Summer Kitchari, 103
Winter Kitchari, 114
Vital essences, 8–9, 20–21

W

Watercress
Creamy Watercress Soup, 123
Spring Pea Salad, 102
Weather, 15
Whey, 112
Carrot Pickle, 185

Winter

Winter
about, 15, 19
meal plan, 47
shopping list, 201
tastes and qualities, 34

Y

Yams
Yam Fries, 150
Yoga, 36
Yogurt
Apricot Tapioca Pudding, 160
Crunchy Yogurt Bowl, 88
Cucumber Raita, 180
Digestive Lassi, 75
Farmer's Cheese Spread, 112
Pistachio Rice with Tahini
Yogurt, 113
Rose Lassi, 76
Sweet Potato Jackets, 157
Yogurt-Dill Dipping Sauce, 182

Z

Zucchini
Flatbread Pizza, 151
Lentil Lasagna, 146–147
Summer Gazpacho, 127

About the Author

LAURA PLUMB is an Ayurvedic practitioner and teacher of Yoga and Jyotish devoted to the Vedic sciences as the supreme teaching on how to live a sacred, sumptuous life. She is the writer and host of the international 58-part TV series *VedaCleanse*, with recipes and daily practices for seasonal wellness, and the host of the 12-part international TV series *Divine Yoga*. Laura teaches and leads retreats internationally plus offers online Seasonal Cleanses and courses on Vedic Wisdom. You can learn more about her at LauraPlumb.com and enjoy her Ayurveda-inspired recipes on her blog: Food-ALoveStory.com.